Beyond Cancer Fatigue

A Path to Reclaiming Energy

Jessa Landmann, ND

WILEY

Published by John Wiley & Sons, Inc., Hoboken, New Jersey.

Library of Congress Cataloging-in-Publication Data has been applied for:

Hardback: 9781394381371
ePDF: 9781394381395
epub: 9781394381388
oBook: 9781394381401

Cover Design: Wiley
Cover Image: Courtesy of Stefan Prodanovic

Brief Contents

Acknowledgments

Thank you to Wiley Publishing for recognizing the importance of this book and for their support, guidance, and resources throughout every stage of its publication.

To my editor, thank you for helping transform my words into a book I'm truly proud of.

To my wonderful children, thank you for your patience and for understanding the time and heart I poured into this book. Your support and loving hearts meant the world to me.

To my amazing friends and loved ones, thank you for your thoughtful feedback and for being the most generous and insightful sounding board I could ask for. Your wisdom and support helped shape this book in countless ways.

And most of all, to my cherished patients—thank you. Thank you for sharing your stories and struggles so openly and for placing your trust in me. Medical school provided the foundation, but my truest education has come from the privilege of working with each of you.

Introduction

The Problem of Cancer-related Fatigue

Imagine a world where "cancer-free" truly means just that—entirely free of cancer and its lingering effects. Imagine completing your treatment, and your doctor telling you that the cancer is gone. The relief is overwhelming, and you begin preparing to resume your life.

Yet, many cancer survivors quickly realize that the end of treatment doesn't necessarily mean the return of energy, clarity, or the life they once knew. You realize you are not quite bouncing back to your old self like you hoped. One of the most debilitating and overlooked after-effects of cancer treatment is cancer-related fatigue (CRF). This persistent exhaustion can linger for months or even years.

CRF is not an ordinary tiredness. It feels like an invisible weight pressing down on your body and mind every day. This type of fatigue is unrelieved by sleep and is often misunderstood, misdiagnosed, or entirely overlooked.

CRF is defined as a "distressing, persistent, subjective sense of tiredness or exhaustion related to cancer or cancer treatment that is not proportional to recent activity and interferes with usual functioning." CRF is a complex and deeply personal challenge.

Cancer survivors often feel there is a disconnect between what they, and those around them, expect they can achieve after treatment, and the realities they face. Even years after treatment, patients report feeling misunderstood by loved ones and doctors who assume life should have returned to normal, and they should be back to feeling like their old selves.

Why dedicate an entire book to fatigue? Fatigue touches every part of our quality of life. Fatigue disrupts focus, drains motivation, and erodes emotional stability. It interferes with work, self-care, and social connection. Many people struggling with CRF become isolated, discouraged, and overwhelmed. It often coexists with depression, pain, and poor sleep, each compounding the other in a vicious cycle.

Beyond Cancer Fatigue: A Path to Reclaiming Energy, First Edition. Jessa Landmann, ND.

But my extensive clinical experience has taught me something powerful: when you begin to address fatigue, everything else starts to improve. Less fatigue means less pain, greater emotional clarity, improved memory, deeper rest, and a renewed interest in the things that bring joy. That's why this book puts fatigue front and center. It's not just a symptom—it's the key to unlocking your well-being.

Another key reason this book focuses on CRF is that it remains one of the most challenging side effects to treat. Despite its prevalence and impact on quality of life, there is no prescription medication specifically designed to address it. As a result, many physicians feel limited in how they can help their patients manage ongoing exhaustion. In addition, some may be unaware of the expanding body of research demonstrating how holistic, lifestyle-based approaches can restore energy and vitality.

As a specialist in integrative oncology, I have seen firsthand that natural and holistic therapies can be remarkably effective in managing CRF. Unlike medication, these approaches address the multiple underlying factors that contribute to fatigue—such as inflammation, hormonal imbalance, nutritional deficiencies, disrupted sleep, and emotional stress.

By targeting the whole person rather than a single symptom, holistic therapies help the body regain balance and resilience. Practices such as acupuncture, gentle exercise, mindfulness, nutrition, and stress-reduction techniques not only alleviate fatigue but also improve mood, sleep quality, and overall well-being. This multidimensional approach allows patients to rebuild their strength from the inside out and reclaim a sense of vitality that conventional medicine alone often cannot provide.

Throughout my practice, I've encountered countless patients who struggle with CRF. Jeanie, a breast cancer survivor, came to me a year after finishing chemotherapy treatment. Despite returning to a healthy diet and routine exercise, she felt mentally foggy, emotionally drained, and deeply exhausted. She tried to return to her life as a mother, teacher, and wife, but her energy never returned to baseline. She was cancer-free but far from feeling free.

In contrast, Mark, a prostate cancer survivor, suffered from an intense fear of recurrence. His fear manifested in extreme social isolation. He felt his friends didn't understand him. Additionally, he felt confused about which foods he should eat and struggled to lose weight. When he came to see me, he recounted his struggles with fatigue and how it impacted his life.

These examples illustrate how CRF can arise from various causes, yet result in similar experiences of fatigue. What will help Jeanie with her energy will be unique from what will help Mark. But how does one figure that out? That's where this book comes in.

With my personal clinical experience in helping cancer survivors to heal, it is clear that fatigue is both a common and a complex experience. We must treat each person's experience of fatigue differently. The true strength of holistic therapies lies in their individualized, whole-person approach to care. Taking a personalized approach to healing means listening deeply to each individual's story of how fatigue manifests in their life, identifying what matters most to them, and tailoring strategies to help them regain control. The path to recovery is never one-size-fits-all.

Consider the contrast between two people complaining of fatigue: one person may be recovering from months of chemotherapy, while another may have had multiple surgeries. Their fatigue may feel similar, but the root causes, and therefore the most effective treatments, are entirely different. Likewise, someone struggling with depression who sleeps excessively will need a different plan than someone who is anxious and sleep deprived.

This book is your roadmap, designed to provide both a clear understanding of CRF and a practical, step-by-step path toward relief. You'll uncover the main factors that drain your energy and learn how to overcome them. By simplifying complex medical insights into practical, relatable strategies, this book empowers you to take control of your health, make meaningful changes and build real, lasting momentum.

Fatigue is not your destiny. There are powerful, research-backed ways to reclaim your strength and energy, and you do not have to face this battle alone. This book will help you not just weather the storm, but bloom in the aftermath.

The Other Side of Fatigue—Energy

Energy—it's something we all experience, yet rarely pause to define. What's truly happening when we feel drained, fatigued, or lacking in vitality? The mystery of energy is not simply a physical matter; it's something that touches our biology, emotions, and even our sense of meaning and purpose.

Our bodies are incredible energy factories, constantly generating the power needed to sustain life. Every heartbeat, every breath, every thought relies on this internal force. But where does this energy come from? Most of us think of energy as something that comes from the food we eat, or something that will appear after a good night's sleep. But anyone struggling with CRF will know this isn't the case.

So what else is at play? Fatigue often has roots that go far deeper than food and sleep alone. While they are a critical piece of the puzzle (which you'll learn about in Chapters 4 and 14), there is a much bigger picture.

Hormones play a vital role. The thyroid, often referred to as the body's "master energy regulator," influences metabolism, mood, digestion, and sleep patterns. If thyroid hormones are low, fatigue is inevitable. The pancreas produces insulin, which helps regulate energy by controlling blood sugar levels and ensuring that our cells receive the fuel they need. Additionally, when sex hormones, like estrogen or testosterone, become imbalanced, they can lead to weight gain, mental fog, night sweats, and disrupted sleep, all of which drain energy.

Energy isn't just about calories, sleep or hormones, though. It's a powerful, multidimensional force that flows through mind and body. There is growing evidence that our thoughts and emotions profoundly influence our physical energy. Consider depression, a condition that doesn't just affect mood but also significantly decreases energy. Cancer survivors dealing with worry, fear, and emotional trauma often find themselves physically exhausted, even without much physical exertion.

These mental and emotional states can manifest as headaches, stomach pain, loss of appetite, and overall fatigue. Neuroscience demonstrates that our thoughts and emotions directly impact how we feel physically, and in this way, can truly wear us down.

This expanded notion of energy reaches far beyond science; it touches the deeper layers of human experience. This broader perspective echoes the timeless wisdom of Chinese medicine and Indian philosophy, both of which view energy as the foundation of life and healing.

In Chinese medicine, this life force is called Qi (pronounced "chee"). Qi flows through pathways in the body, and when it becomes blocked or imbalanced, illness and fatigue often result. Practices such as Tai chi and acupuncture help to balance this Qi and have been shown to reduce cancer-related fatigue.

Similarly, Indian philosophy refers to prana as the vital life force that sustains us. Through breathwork, meditation and yoga, individuals can reconnect with their prana, promoting harmony among the body, mind, and spirit.

These practices are not merely about relaxation; they actively help restore energy and vitality. What these traditions remind us is that energy is not just something we consume or deplete; it's something we can engage with, strengthen, and restore. It's a dynamic force, responsive to how we live, think, feel, and care for ourselves.

In the chapters ahead, we'll take a deeper look at the main factors that contribute to CRF. We'll discuss the physical foundations of healing, such as nutrition, sleep, and exercise, and then explore the mental and emotional dimensions of energy, which are often overlooked in conventional care.

Science tells us that energy can neither be created nor destroyed. Therefore, if you're feeling empty or depleted, the question isn't whether energy still exists. The question should be, where did it go, and more importantly, how can you get it back? This book is here to guide you toward those answers, with compassion, clarity, and practical steps to help you feel like yourself again.

1

Your Journey Starts Here

This book is dedicated to the topic of cancer-related fatigue. All the recommendations made are laser-focused on improving your energy. As you read in the introductory chapter, addressing fatigue requires a holistic and individualized approach. This book is your personalized guide back to vitality.

Attention to a holistic approach is essential. The plan you create will ideally integrate physical health (reducing pain, sleeping better, excellent nutrition, regular physical activity), emotional health (lessening stress, addressing depression and anxiety, taking steps to lower fear of recurrence), and spiritual health (connecting with others, finding meaning for your life, inviting in mindfulness and contemplation).

An emphasis on personalized medicine is also a key point of this book. Truly effective healthcare recognizes that no two individuals are exactly alike, especially when navigating complex health challenges. This is why an individualized approach to medicine isn't just beneficial; it's deemed essential. As you go through this book and read about suggested treatments, choose the ones that match your lifestyle and preferences.

This book is arranged by common side effects that can lead to fatigue. It begins with hormonal changes, including disruptions to thyroid hormones, estrogen, and testosterone. Cancer treatments can drastically lower hormone levels, and these drops can significantly affect energy levels. You'll learn how to manage those side effects to start feeling better.

The following section will delve deeper into the ways your body's metabolism can impact your energy levels. We'll explore common metabolic shifts, including how conditions such as diabetes, unexpected weight gain, and challenges with weight loss can contribute to fatigue.

Following that, we'll shift our focus to the mental and emotional contributors to fatigue. Here, we'll address the profound impact of issues like stress, depression,

Beyond Cancer Fatigue: A Path to Reclaiming Energy, First Edition. Jessa Landmann, ND.

anxiety, and the fear of cancer recurrence on your daily energy. Understanding these connections is crucial for holistic healing.

Finally, you'll discover research-backed complementary therapies to tackle two pervasive energy drainers: insomnia and pain. You'll be equipped with practical strategies to enhance your sleep quality and manage discomfort, allowing you to rediscover the precious rest you need.

Right at the start of each chapter, you'll find a section called "This chapter is for you if...". This helps you quickly identify whether the content directly applies to you, based on your specific cancer type, treatments, and the side effects most impacting your energy. This allows you to effortlessly navigate to what matters most, building a truly customized plan that addresses your individual needs.

To get the most out of what you will read, this book is meant to be interactive. Throughout each chapter, "Reflection Points" invite you to pause, truly absorb what resonates with you, and jot down your insights into a journal. These are your moments to connect the information to your own experience, helping you determine what's relevant and how you can apply it.

The sections called "Clinical Pearls" are where you will find specific, actionable advice, like supplement recommendations and acupuncture protocols. These are direct insights from my own clinical experience, designed to provide you with concrete and powerful tools for your healing journey. Use them to record therapies you're eager to explore, and by the time you reach the end of the book, you'll have organically built your very own, comprehensive fatigue management plan.

You'll also discover "Success Stories" from real patients—individuals I've had the privilege of working with (with names changed, of course). These are genuine survivor stories woven throughout the book, offering comfort, inspiration, and practical ideas for boosting your energy. You'll see firsthand how others have navigated similar challenges and found their path to renewed vitality.

To help you easily synthesize information, many chapters feature flowcharts, infographics, and other visuals to help guide you. And because self-advocacy is paramount, you'll find sections called "For Your Healthcare Practitioner." These are designed to be shared directly with your doctors, empowering you to confidently discuss specific assessments, blood tests, or complementary therapies that could further support your energy and well-being.

Throughout your reading, you will discover that you no longer need to follow generic advice that doesn't consider individual circumstances or acknowledge advancements in research. While reading, you will encounter actionable and impactful solutions. You will be equipped with self-advocacy tools to foster a sense of empowerment and gain knowledge about complementary treatments, ensuring you address all your needs.

The solutions in this book are practical, easy to implement, and, where possible, treatments you can do yourself. Some therapies, such as acupuncture or massage, may require professional assistance. However, if certain resources are unavailable, multiple treatment options are suggested to you that can suit your preferences and individual situation.

To help assure you that you are in the right place to address cancer-related fatigue, here are some frequently asked questions.

How Can I Get the Most Out of This Book?

This book is your personal toolkit, designed to help you create a customized fatigue management plan that truly fits your unique experiences and ongoing challenges. To make it even easier, remember those helpful sections at the start of each chapter, "This chapter is for you if...." They'll help you quickly see if a chapter is relevant to your unique situation right now, allowing you to focus on what you need most and even skip sections for the time being.

For example, if you're a woman who hasn't experienced significant weight gain, you might consider skipping chapters focused on testosterone or specific weight loss methods. But try not to skip too much! You may uncover unexpected insights into the root causes of your fatigue in other chapters. You may be tempted to bypass the chapter on diabetes, but you'll learn that it's quite common for cancer survivors to develop insulin resistance, which can lead to pre-diabetes and diabetes, which is important to rule out.

Feel empowered to begin with the chapters that resonate most with you at this moment. Then, whenever you feel ready for more insight and guidance, the other chapters will be waiting to support you further on your journey to renewed energy.

I'm Afraid of Getting My Hopes Up, as Nothing I've Tried in the Past Has Worked. How Can I Be Sure I'll Feel Better?

Medicine is not a one-size-fits-all field. The advice you've received in the past or the approaches you've tried based on other information might not be suited specifically to you. Additionally, some factors could be affecting your ability to regain energy.

- Relying solely on rest—many people might think that rest alone will alleviate their fatigue, leading to frustration.
- Not being proactive—many cancer survivors are told to "give it time" and that their energy will improve on its own. This is often not the case. Healing is a proactive, not a passive, process.

- Over-reliance on caffeine—some turn to coffee or other energy drinks, which may lead to a temporary increase in energy, only to lead to a crash.
- Ignoring your mental and emotional health—focusing only on physical solutions without addressing mental health can leave underlying issues unresolved, perpetuating fatigue.
- Giving up too soon—this can be detrimental, as recovering energy can take some time. Additionally, some treatments recommended in this book may take several weeks or even a few months to take effect. Sticking with it is key!

As you read in the opening of this chapter, this book aims to provide you with a personalized system to develop a fatigue management plan. This approach to fatigue is unique and is probably unlike anything you have encountered before. Furthermore, the treatments recommended in the book are all evidence-based, meaning there is scientific support to show that the treatments you try will be effective.

Are There Specific Foods or Diets That Can Help Reduce My Fatigue?

Absolutely! Nutrition is one of the key pillars for boosting energy. There has been extensive research on the connection between nutrition, cancer, and fatigue. Nutrition can be a very confusing subject for cancer survivors, as it seems like everything they read online is contradictory. This is precisely why this book has dedicated significant space to the topic of nutrition.

You will not only learn about a fatigue-reduction eating style, but also how to lower your risk of recurrence using food as medicine. Additionally, we will break down and analyze fad diets and recommend specific eating patterns that boost your energy levels while avoiding those that may leave you feeling drained. Chapter 4 will teach you all you need to know about food!

Are There Any Supplements That Could Help Me with My Energy Levels?

Yes! Supplements can be used to address various health concerns related to fatigue. There are herbal therapies that improve mental and emotional issues, such as anxiety and depression. Some supplements can help you achieve deeper, more restorative sleep, while others can help reduce pain levels. Additionally, there are supplements that can help alleviate hot flashes in both men and women, as well as supplements designed to lower blood sugar and support muscle growth.

Supplements are part of a holistic approach to managing fatigue and can sometimes be an excellent addition to other lifestyle changes, such as exercise and a balanced diet. The supplements recommended in this book are supported by scientific research and are generally considered safe.

How Can I Communicate My Fatigue to My Doctors?

It's incredibly common for cancer patients to experience fatigue, and it's equally common to feel unheard or unsure how to talk about it with your doctors. Many patients want to explore this topic, only to find their healthcare team dismissive or uninformed. The good news is that there are practical ways to have more effective and open dialogues.

The first step in discussing fatigue is to inform your doctor beforehand that you have specific concerns and require extra time during the appointment. Make sure this conversation isn't rushed.

The second step in effective communication is to make your experience clear. Fatigue isn't just "being tired"; it's a complex, often debilitating symptom that needs to be taken seriously. Start a diary where you track your daily activities and symptoms, writing down specifically how fatigue impacts you, and rate your energy on a scale of 1–10.

Instead of just saying, "I'm tired," describe how it affects your life.

- I used to be able to walk around the block, but now I get exhausted after just a few steps.
- I'm so exhausted that I can't concentrate on my favorite book or hold a conversation.
- My fatigue sometimes prevents me from performing basic chores, such as cooking or showering.
- I'm sleeping 10 hours a night but still feel like I haven't slept at all.

In the journal, record these experiences for several days or a week before your appointment, and note any times of day when your energy is higher or lower. This provides your doctor with concrete data, not just general complaints. Link your energy levels to other issues like pain, insomnia, anxiety, or depression. "My joint pain keeps me awake, and then the lack of sleep makes my fatigue unbearable."

If you feel your concerns are being brushed aside, be persistent, but polite, reiterating their importance. "I understand we've focused on my cancer treatment in the past, but this fatigue is significantly impacting my ability to cope and affecting my quality of life. What steps can we take to address it?"

My Doctor Does Not Believe in Holistic Therapies, or Says They Don't Have Any Knowledge About Them. How Can I Get My Doctor's Support?

Many doctors, including those in conventional oncology, may not be experts in holistic therapies. Their primary focus is often on treating the cancer itself, and this topic is not usually part of their training. Here's how you can approach the conversation effectively.

First, be receptive to their concerns. They may have valid reasons for caution due to possible drug interactions or your particular health situation. This should be a dialogue, not a debate. If they voice concerns, ask, "What are your specific concerns about this therapy for me?" or "What would you recommend instead for this symptom?"

Second, where possible, show them published research or practice guidelines. You could begin with the joint guidelines from the American Society of Clinical Oncology and the Society for Integrative Oncology (ASCO/SIO). These are reputable medical organizations that offer recommendations for fatigue and pain. This book also includes hundreds of references, so if you find something you'd like to share with your doctor, they can look up the references to learn more.

Third, use the terms "holistic," "complementary," or "integrative" when describing treatments. Avoid the use of "alternative" therapy. Emphasize that you see these therapies as complementary to your care, that you remain fully committed to conventional health care, but are seeking additional ways to support your body and manage side effects.

And fourth, if your primary oncology team is consistently dismissive and you strongly wish to explore these options, consider consulting with an integrative oncologist or a naturopathic doctor experienced in oncology. They can collaborate with the rest of your healthcare team. The Oncology Association of Naturopathic Physicians maintains a list of doctors across North America who specialize in integrative oncology.

Having these conversations takes courage and preparation, but advocating for your full well-being is a crucial part of your cancer journey.

How Do I Balance My Everyday Responsibilities with Taking Time for Myself to Heal, Without Feeling Guilty?

Cancer survivors often navigate a complex emotional landscape, and among the most challenging feelings is guilt. This guilt can manifest when trying to prioritize self-care, manage time, and set boundaries, especially after a life-altering experience like cancer. It's a natural response to having faced a significant challenge.

Cancer survivors may experience guilt for several reasons:

- Survivor's guilt—this is a feeling of guilt for surviving when others may not have, or for having different outcomes. This can lead to a sense of obligation to "make the most" of life, often by overextending oneself.
- Feeling like a burden—feeling that you were or are a burden to loved ones during treatment may lead to a desire to "make it up" to them by doing more than you can realistically manage.
- Loss of identity—this can feel like a struggle to reconcile the "old you" (who might have been highly independent or a primary caregiver) with the "new you" (who may have different physical or emotional capacities). This can lead to guilt over not meeting past expectations.
- Societal expectations—this can be a subtle or overt societal pressure to "bounce back" quickly and be perpetually grateful, which can make it difficult to acknowledge limitations or express needs.

These sources of guilt can lead to the feeling that you must return to life as usual, continuing all the activities you used to do and perhaps even more. This may cause additional guilt about taking time for yourself. Reducing the grip of guilt requires a shift in perspective, along with practical strategies for managing your energy and relationships.

First, when it comes to taking the time for self-care, you should reframe it as treatment, not a treat. Start viewing self-care (including rest, healthy eating, gentle exercise, and emotional processing) as an integral part of your recovery and ongoing health management, just like medication or follow-up appointments. It's nonnegotiable for sustaining your well-being.

Second, explain to yourself, and perhaps to others, that by taking care of yourself, you are increasing your capacity to be present and engaged in the ways that truly matter. You can't pour from an empty cup. Remind yourself that prioritizing your health now helps prevent potential burnout down the line.

Third, treat yourself like a friend. We are often much kinder to others than we are to ourselves. Ask yourself, "If my closest friend were going through what I am, what advice would I give them? Would I tell them to push themselves until they collapse, or would I encourage rest and gentle care?"

Next, when it comes to taking on new responsibilities or continuing with your old way of life, communicate your "new normal." Your capacity has likely changed, so be honest with yourself and others about your current energy levels and limitations. You don't need to justify or over-explain. Try direct statements like, "I appreciate you asking, but I don't have the energy for that right now." Or, "I can commit to [small task] but won't be able to do [larger task]."

Understand that others may have unrealistic expectations. However, it's not your job to constantly meet them. You are allowed to protect your peace and your health. As well, you should value your presence. Your greatest contribution to loved ones might now be your calm presence, your shared laughter, or simply your continued existence, rather than constant "doing." Remind yourself of this every day.

And finally, consider professional help. A therapist or counsellor specializing in cancer survivorship can provide tools and strategies for navigating guilt, processing trauma, and building healthier coping mechanisms.

Lessening the guilt isn't an overnight process, but it's a vital part of thriving after cancer. By shifting your perspective, practicing self-compassion, setting firm boundaries, and prioritizing your well-being above all else, you can cultivate a life that truly supports your healing and allows you to live with greater peace and energy.

Hopefully, these initial answers have brought you clarity and a sense of reassurance that this book can truly help you. This book is, indeed, designed to be your steadfast companion in overcoming fatigue. Now, prepare to embark on a transformative journey. With your journal in hand, let's delve into the powerful strategies and insights that await you.

2

Decoding Your Fatigue: Why Am I So Tired

The greater the obstacle, the more glory in overcoming it

—Moliere

Cancer-related fatigue (CRF) is far more than just being tired. It's an overwhelming exhaustion that stubbornly refuses to lift, no matter how much you rest. Unlike the fatigue that fades with a good night's sleep, CRF has deep roots in the cancer itself, the powerful treatments used to fight it, and the side effects and aftermath of those treatments.

Cancer places immense demands on your body. Your immune system works overtime to fight it, and your body feels the desire to give in to that fight. In addition, essential therapies like chemotherapy, radiation, immunotherapy, and surgery can trigger widespread inflammation and blood loss and disrupt your cells' vital functions. All of these factors conspire to deplete your energy reserves.

After treatment, people are left with the fallout of such an intense experience, and in addition to the physical toll on the body, the emotional toll wreaks havoc. It's crucial to understand that CRF is a very real, physically and emotionally rooted condition. It is absolutely not a sign of weakness, laziness, or a lack of willpower. You are not imagining it, and you are certainly not alone in experiencing it.

Understanding the true causes of your fatigue can be incredibly empowering. The aim in sharing this information is never to lay blame if other conditions are present, but rather to release you from any self-blame or guilt, paving a clearer path toward healing. Feeling guilty only adds to the burden, making you feel responsible for feeling unwell.

If any of the following information resonates with you, use it as a powerful insight. The goal is to pinpoint exactly what's standing in your way of feeling better and then channel your energy into recovery. Start making a list of what clicks for you, and we'll explore how to tackle each of these challenges with practical, evidence-informed strategies.

Beyond Cancer Fatigue: A Path to Reclaiming Energy, First Edition. Jessa Landmann, ND.

REFLECTION POINT
Start a journal or personal notebook. While going through the next section, make a list of any factors that may be contributing to your energy depletion. Use this as a living record that we'll return to while going through the rest of the book.

The 3P Model of Fatigue

The 3P model helps explain the different layers of CRF. It breaks fatigue down into three main contributors:

1. Predisposing factors—what was already present before cancer.
2. Precipitating factors—what cancer and its treatments have done to the body.
3. Perpetuating factors—what contributes to fuel fatigue over time.

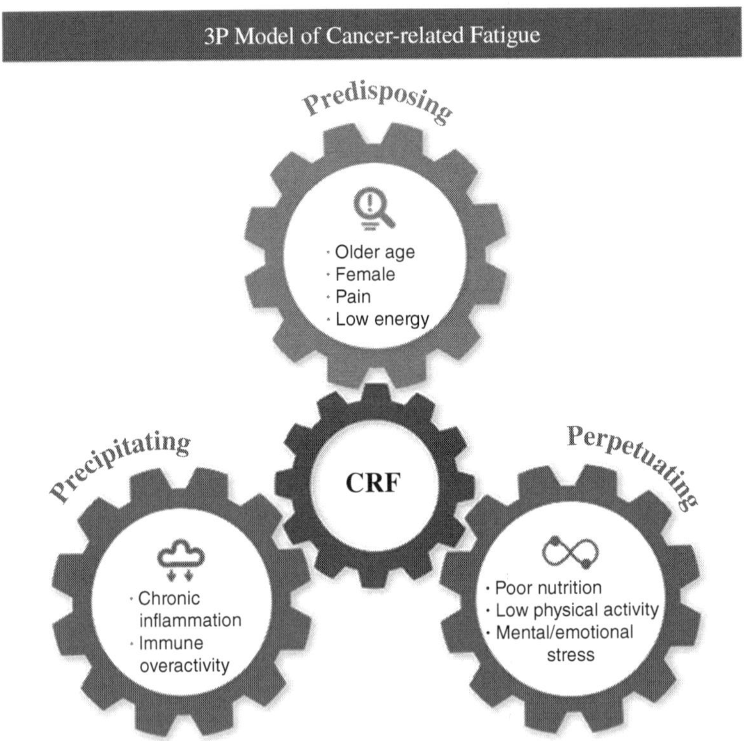

Predisposing Factors (Things That Were Already There Before Cancer)

Some factors are beyond your control, such as your age or biological sex. However, older individuals tend to report more severe fatigue, and women are twice as likely as men to develop moderate to severe CRF [1].

If you experienced fatigue before your cancer diagnosis, you are more likely to continue struggling with chronic fatigue long after your treatment is over. Pre-existing fatigue is the strongest predictor of long-term CRF [2]. Other physical symptoms, such as a low appetite, drowsiness, pain, or shortness of breath, can compound the problem, predisposing someone to persistent fatigue.

Inflammation is another key factor. Individuals with higher inflammation markers prior to treatment are significantly more likely to experience fatigue long-term [3].

Your mental and emotional state also plays a role. People with depression and anxiety tend to experience higher levels of fatigue. Moreover, even without a formal diagnosis, thought patterns such as sadness, self-criticism, and irritability can exacerbate tiredness. Behaviors such as catastrophizing, all-or-nothing thinking, and avoidance further contribute [4].

Here are some examples of how someone might think in these situations:

- Catastrophizing—"I have cancer. I'm going to die."
- All-or-nothing thinking—"Because I got cancer, my body must be completely broken."
- Avoidant behaviors—"I'm afraid of bad news, so I won't go to my follow-up scans."

In Chapter 1, we examined how our thoughts can drain our energy. Negative thinking patterns can lead to low energy and fatigue. Identifying them is the first step, as they can offer a powerful opportunity for change.

REFLECTION POINT
Take a moment to write down any recurring thoughts you've had lately. Are they positive and hopeful? Or do they weigh you down? Do you have more negative thoughts than positive ones? How do they make you feel physically?

Precipitating Factors (What Treatment and Cancer Did to You)

The most common ways cancer is treated are surgery, chemotherapy, immunotherapy, and radiation. They damage cancer cells, but they also harm healthy tissues. That collateral damage triggers inflammation and disturbs the body's delicate internal balance, resulting in the side effects you experience, notably fatigue.

Inflammation and an Overactive Immune System

In simple terms, inflammation is the body's natural and necessary response to healing. Think of inflammation like an emergency response team. When something goes wrong, whether you've cut your finger, caught a cold, or suffered a more serious injury, your body immediately springs into action.

It starts by calling in reinforcements. This is where the immune system steps in. Much like a home security system, the immune system detects threats and sends out alerts to protect the body. You may notice a fever, body aches, or a reduced appetite, which are signs that your immune system is mobilizing. Blood vessels widen to deliver oxygen and nutrients to the affected area, which is why you may feel a sensation of heat or notice redness. Swelling acts like a cushion, protecting the injured area while the body's "repair crews" begin the healing process.

Inflammation is at the core of many side effects experienced during and after cancer treatment. It disrupts sleep, contributes to pain, reduces appetite, causes brain fog, and profoundly drains energy. If you've ever had the flu, you've likely felt more than just fever and body aches; you probably also felt exhausted. That's inflammation at work, urging your body to slow down and recover.

However, sometimes this internal "emergency crew" doesn't stand down, even after the initial crisis has passed. When inflammation persists after it's no longer needed, it becomes chronic, and that's when problems can become long-lasting. The immune system not only sounds the alarm and mobilizes healing, but it's also supposed to know when to switch off. When it doesn't, long-term fatigue and other lingering symptoms can set in.

Two systems in the body are susceptible to chronic inflammation: your muscles' mitochondria and your brain. Damage in either of these areas plays a significant role in CRF.

Inflammation of the Mitochondria

Mitochondria are often described as the "powerhouse" of the cell, as they generate most of the energy your body uses to function. But when mitochondrial function is impaired, energy production slows down dramatically. This is what happens after harsh treatments like chemotherapy, which produce toxins that interfere with the function of the mitochondria. It's a bit like running your car on empty.

Muscle cells are very sensitive to this kind of damage; when mitochondria in the muscles are affected, it leads to muscle loss, weakness, and fatigue [5]. That's why even simple tasks, such as standing up to get a glass of water, can feel exhausting.

Inflammation of the Brain

The brain is susceptible to inflammation. When inflamed, you might experience symptoms like low appetite, depression, mental fog, and problems thinking.

Inflammation in the brain can also reduce blood flow and interrupt the delivery of essential nutrients, making it more difficult to think clearly and regulate emotions. We understand that chemotherapy crosses into the brain, which may result in direct damage to the cells of the brain, and even impair the growth of new cells [6].

CRF is a specific type of fatigue that results from a combination of muscle dysfunction, inflammation, and brain toxicity. You're not stuck with it. While these processes are complex, they're not impossible to address. The upcoming chapters will walk you through practical strategies to help restore energy by repairing the damage that inflammation leaves behind.

REFLECTION POINT
Take a moment to reflect: Are you experiencing muscle weakness, brain fog, or problems thinking clearly? Jot down what you've noticed in your journal. The more you understand your symptoms, the more effectively you can begin building a personalized recovery plan.

Perpetuating Factors (Things That Keep the Fatigue Going)

Perpetuating factors are related to lifestyle and mood, particularly nutrition, physical activity, and mental/emotional stress. Individuals with low levels of physical activity often experience more severe fatigue. Many cancer survivors assume that rest is the best way to restore energy. While rest is important, too much inactivity can actually worsen fatigue. Our bodies are built to move, and gentle, regular physical activity helps improve blood flow, muscle strength, sleep quality, and even mood.

Nutrition is another major player. Fatigue often worsens when the body isn't getting the fuel it needs, particularly protein. In cancer survivors, low protein intake is commonly linked to persistent fatigue. Protein supports muscle repair, immune function, and hormone production, all of which are critical to recovery. Increasing protein intake can be one of the most reliable and immediate ways to boost energy.

People battling or recovering from cancer feel like they are on an emotional roller coaster. The emotions that accompany constant fatigue can be a crazy ride of ups and downs. Anxiety creeps in. Will I ever feel like myself again? Will I be able to do what I used to love? These questions can evoke frustration, fear, and sadness. You may find yourself withdrawing from others, feeling misunderstood, or even resentful. Over time, these emotions can lead to low self-esteem, loss of confidence, and a deep sense of mental exhaustion.

Recognizing the emotional component of fatigue can be a turning point. It allows space for self-compassion. It invites others to gain a better understanding of what you're going through. And it opens the door to healing not just your body but your whole self.

Final Thoughts

CRF can be relentless and can cast a long shadow over someone, significantly impacting their quality of life. The emotional and physical weariness that comes with the task of overcoming utter exhaustion can leave someone feeling isolated, misunderstood, withdrawn, and struggling to connect with the world around them.

The 3P model of fatigue identifies physical and emotional factors that contribute to fatigue. These factors interact in a complex manner and often influence one another. The following chapters will guide you through strategies to lower inflammation, fuel your body with energy-boosting nutrition, support brain and muscle recovery, and develop a personalized movement plan.

In addition, the book will address other causes of low energy that have not been discussed yet, such as hormonal imbalances, changes in weight, and pain management. You will receive a comprehensive roadmap, not just to survive fatigue but to rise above it, step by step.

For Healthcare Practitioners: Screening and Assessment

Despite being impaired by fatigue, many patients may assume it is simply a natural part of their illness and that there is nothing they can do about it. Therefore, they may not be able to raise their concerns with healthcare practitioners. It is the duty and responsibility of healthcare practitioners to provide information about fatigue, assess symptoms at baseline, and screen for them consistently throughout treatment and survivorship. This recommendation is supported by guidelines from the U.S. National Comprehensive Cancer Network (NCCN), the Canadian Association of Psychosocial Oncology (CAPO), and the European Society for Medical Oncology (ESMO) [7].

A recent survey of 2,508 patients found that 41% did not recall ever being asked by their treating physician about fatigue or exhaustion. Among those who were asked, fatigue was addressed less frequently in older adults compared to patients under the age of 70 [8].

This may be due to a lack of awareness among clinicians. A survey of 400 oncologists and 400 oncology nurses revealed that many underestimated both the prevalence and the clinical significance of CRF [9].

In light of these findings, it's clear that CRF is a significant yet often overlooked challenge for many patients, and a gap remains between the experiences of patients and the awareness and interventions of healthcare providers. Closing this gap requires a concerted effort: patients need to feel empowered to voice their struggles, and crucially, healthcare practitioners must actively inquire about, assess, and address CRF throughout every stage of the cancer journey. While this book is intended for survivors of cancer struggling to regain their energy, as a healthcare professional, you will gain valuable knowledge about this important subject.

Blood Work

To evaluate inflammation, the standard markers are erythrocyte sedimentation rate (ESR) and C-reactive protein (CRP). Ample research links elevated CRP levels with fatigue.

To evaluate nutritional deficiencies, routine testing of albumin, vitamin B12, and folate is recommended. Albumin is a useful indicator of protein status, and increasing dietary protein is an effective way to boost albumin levels [10].

To evaluate anemia, especially anemia of chronic disease, ferritin, transferrin saturation, and ESR should be measured, along with a complete blood cell count.

To evaluate thyroid function, a comprehensive thyroid panel (TSH, free T4, free T3, anti-TPO, and anti-TG) is necessary to rule out thyroid disease and subclinical hypothyroidism.

To evaluate insulin resistance, fasting insulin and fasting blood glucose are needed to calculate the HOMA-IR score. Continuous glucose monitoring is also helpful to determine how blood sugar levels change in response to specific foods, which can inform personalized nutrition advice.

And finally, a 4-point cortisol test is ideal for determining how cortisol levels fluctuate throughout the day. At the very least, morning cortisol levels should be ordered as part of a comprehensive evaluation for causes of CRF.

References

1 Hoffman AJ, von Eye A, Gift AG, et al. Testing a theoretical model of perceived self-efficacy for cancer-related fatigue self-management and optimal physical functional status. Nurs Res, 2009; 58:32–41.

2 Susanne K, Michael F, Thomas S, et al. Predictors of fatigue in cancer patients: a longitudinal study. Support Care Cancer, 2019; 27:3463–3471.

3 Di Meglio A, Havas J, Pagliuca M, et al. A bio-behavioral model of systemic inflammation at breast cancer diagnosis and fatigue of clinical importance two years later. Ann Oncol, 2024; 35(11):1048–1060.

4 Hughes A, Suleman S, Rimes KA, et al. Cancer-related fatigue and functional impairment—towards an understanding of cognitive and behavioural factors. J Psychosom Res, 2020; 134:110127.

5 Yang S, Chu S, Gao Y, et al. A narrative review of cancer-related fatigue (CRF) and its possible pathogenesis. Cells, 2019; 8:738.

6 Rao V, Bhutan R, Kumari P, et al. Chapter two—chemobrain: a review on mechanistic insight, targets and treatments. Adv Canc Res, 2022; 155:29–76.

7 Fabi A, Bhargava R, Fatigoni S, et al. Cancer related fatigue: ESMO Clinical Practice Guidelines for diagnosis and treatment. Ann Oncol, 2020; 31(6):713–723.

8 Schmidt ME, Bergbold S, Hermann S, et al. Knowledge, perceptions and management of cancer related fatigue; the patients' perspective. Support Care Cancer, 2021; 29:2063–2071.

9 Williams LA, Bohac C, Hunter S, et al. Patient and health care provider perceptions of cancer related fatigue and pain. Support Care Cancer, 2016; 24(10):4357–4363.

10 Ghoshal A, Damani A, Muckten M. Association of cancer related fatigue with other symptoms and impact on quality of life of palliative care patients in a tertiary cancer institute: a prospective observational study. J Pain Symptom Manage, 2016; 51:435.

Part I

Foundational Treatments for Cancer-related Fatigue

3

Your Starter Kit: Practical Strategies for Everyone

Energy and persistence conquer all things

—Benjamin Franklin

This chapter is for you if:

- You wish to start exploring complementary therapies that can help you feel better, and you can begin right away.
- You are curious about a general overview of evidence-based treatments that have been shown to help reduce fatigue.

Understanding Your Unique Path to Healing

Cancer-related fatigue (CRF) is a multifaceted condition resulting from various factors. That's why the most effective approaches to healing are just as varied and need to be tailored to you. Proper lasting recovery comes from a personalized plan rooted in three key areas:

1. Your cancer journey: considering the specific treatments you've received in the past.
2. Your current challenges: identifying lingering side effects, such as pain or sleep disturbances.
3. Your overall health: recognizing other conditions you may be managing, like high blood pressure or diabetes.

Beyond Cancer Fatigue: A Path to Reclaiming Energy, First Edition. Jessa Landmann, ND.

This kind of individualized care is ideal, but it can be challenging to access in today's overburdened healthcare system. Doctors and nurses, despite their dedication, may not have the time for fully personalized planning. That's why *general recommendations* are so valuable, as they provide a helpful starting point, no matter your history or current health needs.

Finding What Resonates with You

Beyond medical advice, your interests and what feels right for your body play a significant role in successful healing. In the following sections, we'll explore a variety of complementary and mind–body therapies. Remember, what works for one person may not work for another. Some may find solace and energy in physical activity, while others may find therapy helpful, and for some, a simple supplement might offer the most relief. Your healing journey should align with your unique preferences and bring meaning to your recovery.

Trusted Guidance for Your Recovery

The recommendations in this chapter are based on guidelines from two respected organizations: the American Society of Clinical Oncology (ASCO) and the Society for Integrative Oncology (SIO). These groups are dedicated to comprehensive cancer care, focusing on research, education, and promoting the highest quality patient experience. In 2024, they collaboratively published a practice guideline specifically for managing fatigue in adult cancer survivors, offering a valuable, evidence-based starting point [1]. While these clinical guidelines provide a broad approach, they're invaluable when you're unsure where to start.

The ASCO/SIO guideline is based on a thorough review of research into complementary therapies. Their recommendations are organized by the strength of the evidence. A treatment marked "should" means there is strong support from high-quality research. A "may" recommendation means the evidence is promising, though not as conclusive. In both cases, the benefits of these treatments are considered to outweigh potential risks.

The following table summarizes these expert recommendations for managing CRF, both during and after active treatment.

Recommendation	Strength	Explanation	Active or posttreatment
Combination of aerobic exercise plus resistance training	Should	There are great benefits of physical activity for CRF. The intensity of the exercise should be based on patient preference, likelihood of adherence, and safety.	Active and Post
Cognitive behavioral therapy (CBT)	Should	CBT is a well-validated therapy for fatigue and can be delivered in person, virtually, and with or without hypnosis.	Active and Post
Mindfulness-based stress reduction	Should	Interventions are commonly weekly sessions for 8–12 weeks in length.	Active and Post
Tai chi	Should	Sessions ranged from 20 to 60 minutes, 3–5 times per week.	Active
Ginseng	May	This traditional herb is safe, and doses of 2,000–3,000 mg per day were found to be most effective.	Active
Yoga	May	Generally considered safe, and participants can choose their intensity levels.	Post
Acupressure or acupuncture	May	Interventions are commonly six weeks in duration but may be longer in length.	Post

These recommendations are designed as a safe and practical starting point for patients and their families. They do not require lab tests, and they carry minimal risk. Let's now explore each one in more detail.

Exercise—Cardio and Resistance Training

For many cancer survivors, the path to regaining energy can feel long and challenging. But there's a powerful, often overlooked tool that can make a real difference: exercise. This isn't just about building strength or improving fitness; it's about rewiring your body's energy system. Engaging in regular physical activity sparks a cascade of beneficial changes, from boosting blood flow and oxygen delivery to your cells to releasing your body's natural mood elevators and pain relievers.

It strengthens your muscles, clears your mind, and promotes deeper sleep—all critical factors in combating the persistent grip of fatigue.

"Cardio" refers to activities that increase your heart rate and breathing, such as swimming, brisk walking, or hiking. These exercises get your heart and lungs working harder, often leaving you warm, sweaty, and a bit breathless. Although that sensation can be uncomfortable at first, the benefits are substantial.

Resistance training, commonly referred to as weightlifting, is one of the most effective methods for building strength and increasing muscle mass. It also increases your heart rate, providing cardiovascular benefits. Forget the idea that cardio must mean hours on a treadmill—lifting weights can be just as effective, and far more enjoyable.

One reason resistance training is emphasized is that muscle, an often overlooked organ system, plays a crucial role in overall health. Muscle mass naturally declines by 3–8% per decade after the age of 30, and the rate of decline accelerates after the age of 60 [2]. Research consistently shows that maintaining muscle mass is one of the strongest predictors of longevity and healthy aging. Because building muscle is so important, Chapter 18 teaches you how to get started.

Strong muscles help prevent falls, improve balance, and even support cognitive health. One study linked lower muscle strength and slower walking speed with cognitive decline [3]. A systematic review of 47 studies also found that physical inactivity significantly increases the risk of dementia [4].

Taking care of your muscles isn't just about aesthetics and looking stronger; it's about protecting your future vitality and long-term well-being.

For cancer survivors struggling with fatigue, resistance training offers a powerful, multi-layered solution. Low muscle mass, physical inactivity, and cognitive impairment are all closely linked to persistent fatigue. The encouraging news? Resistance training can simultaneously target and improve all of these processes. It's a comprehensive strategy that empowers you to rebuild strength, sharpen your mind, and diminish fatigue, all in one go.

Success Story

Lisa, a breast cancer survivor, had completed both radiation and chemotherapy. Before her diagnosis, she was very active, as she and her husband used to work out at home six days a week. Lisa also loved swimming and described her pre-cancer energy as a solid 10 out of 10. A year after treatment, however, she rated it at a 7 out of 10.

To some, a 7/10 might sound high. But for Lisa, it felt like a loss. She began therapy to process the idea that she might never feel fully like herself again. When we assessed her body composition, we found that her muscle mass was significantly below average for her height and age, despite her normal weight. I encouraged her to rebuild muscle, explaining that doing so could very well bring her energy back to a 10.

Lisa resumed weight training with her husband. After just one month, she gained 1.5 pounds of muscle. She admitted that many days she did not feel like working out, but she committed to training three days a week so she would not feel too exhausted. She achieved this with the love and encouragement of her partner.

Three months later, after consistent strength training with gradually increasing weights, she rated her energy at 9.5 out of 10.

Cognitive Behavioral Therapy

CBT is a valuable tool in managing CRF. It focuses on the connection among thoughts, feelings, behaviors, and fatigue, and then aims to help people identify and shift negative patterns to improve their energy. Research is both strong and encouraging, making it one of the most practical and effective strategies available.

The recommendation of this book is to seek out an experienced therapist with whom you can build a strong, supportive relationship. However, if a therapist is not accessible to you, there are apps such as BetterHelp and Talkspace that can be more cost-effective and convenient. There are also many self-help workbooks that you could access and work through.

While this book is not a CBT manual, it can serve as a starting point to help you explore CBT techniques that can improve your energy. Let's explore some concepts that can be beneficial and put into practice today.

Activity Management and Pacing

Activity management and pacing involve breaking down tasks into smaller, manageable steps and scheduling rest periods throughout the day to maintain optimal performance. These strategies help prevent what's known as a "boom-bust" cycle. In this pattern, someone experiences a burst of energy, only to overexert themselves, resulting in a significant energy crash that can last for several days afterwards. CBT helps individuals to recognize their limits and plan their activities accordingly.

It's essential to resist the temptation to do everything on a "good day." Even if you feel great and want to mow the lawn, clean the house, and run errands all in one day, please don't. Focus on one or two tasks a day, even when your energy feels high. This approach helps restore a sense of control and predictability, preventing the highs and lows that often accompany CRF.

REFLECTION POINT

Create a master to-do list encompassing everything you need to accomplish. Please don't hold back; get it all down on paper. From that comprehensive list, select just one or two tasks you will commit to completing each day. Place these specific tasks on your daily calendar. By doing this, you're not just making a list; you're creating a realistic and manageable plan that frees your mind from the burden of constant worry. Commit to feeling a sense of accomplishment and progress.

Cognitive Restructuring

One of the initial steps in cognitive restructuring is recognizing negative thoughts. CRF can cause negative thoughts and beliefs, such as "I'll never have any energy again" or "I'm useless." CBT helps individuals recognize these negative thoughts and question their accuracy.

A good technique to manage these negative thoughts is called thought stopping. When you catch yourself thinking poorly about yourself, say out loud, "stop!" From there, you can then ask yourself follow-up questions, such as "Is it true that I'm useless?" and "Is it true that I'll never have energy again?"

Another way to challenge negative thoughts is to examine the evidence for and against them and develop a more realistic and balanced perspective. For example, instead of thinking "I'm useless," someone might learn to think, "I'm experiencing fatigue, but I still accomplish things at my own pace. That's enough, and I'm proud of myself."

REFLECTION POINT

Create a list of positive affirmations that you can keep handy to read aloud and repeat to yourself. Positive affirmations should be in the present tense, be about you, and only contain positive, uplifting language. Make these affirmations personal and meaningful. For example, "I'm healing from cancer and am learning to empower myself," "I am strong mentally and soon will feel strong physically," or "I am stronger than my challenges and can overcome anything."

Problem-solving Skills

CBT also helps people develop skills to break down large problems into smaller, more manageable problems. When CRF leads to feelings of overwhelm, structured problem-solving techniques can be incredibly valuable. Here's a simple way to begin:

- Define the Problem Clearly
  Identify the specific challenge that is causing you stress. Instead of saying "I'm overwhelmed," try to pinpoint what's causing that feeling. Is it a

mountain of housework? Too many medical appointments? Demands by, or responsibilities for, other family members?

- Brainstorm Solutions
  Generate a list of possible solutions and consider the resources available to you. Can some appointments be done via telehealth? Can you delegate some of your other responsibilities to other family members? For cleaning tasks, break them down into smaller tasks. For example, instead of thinking "I have to clean my whole house," see it as cleaning one sink in the morning, dusting one shelf in the afternoon, and polishing one mirror in the evening.
- Create an Action Plan
  Use organizational tools such as calendars or to-do lists. Remember to be flexible and adjust your plan if it's not working out as planned. Focus on one small step at a time, and don't try to do everything at once. Most importantly, practice self-compassion and communicate with your loved ones.

Mindfulness-based Interventions

Mindfulness has gained popularity thanks to the works of several notable pioneers, including Deepak Chopra and Jon Kabat-Zinn. If you are unfamiliar with their books, they are highly recommended as a good starting point to familiarize yourself with this topic.

At its core, mindfulness is the practice of paying attention to the present moment without judgment or criticism. It's about cultivating a nonreactive awareness of your thoughts, feelings, body sensations, and the external environment. Rather than getting swept away by tidal waves of your thoughts—anxieties about the future, regrets about the past—mindfulness teaches you to observe them as they are. It's not about suppressing thoughts: it's about acknowledging their presence without getting entangled in them.

One of the primary ways mindfulness helps to combat fatigue is by reducing the body's response to stress. After a cancer diagnosis, many people experience depression, anxiety, and fear of recurrence, all of which cause stress. Stress activates the sympathetic nervous system, also known as the "fight or flight" response, which triggers the release of the stress hormone cortisol. When stress and cortisol remain elevated for prolonged periods, sleep disturbances, weakened immune function, and exhaustion ensue. A regular mindfulness practice has been shown to lower cortisol levels, enhance mood, improve sleep quality, and increase energy levels [5].

There are many simple ways to bring mindfulness into your daily life. One straightforward technique is mindful breathing. When worry begins to rise, find a quiet spot where you can sit comfortably. Close your eyes and turn your attention to your breath. Notice how the air feels as it enters your nose and expands your chest. Breathe in for a count of five, and exhale for a count of five. Deep, slow breathing activates our parasympathetic nervous system, which is the part of the nervous system responsible for calming the body and mind.

Another way to incorporate mindfulness is through body scans. We can do this daily to check for areas of tension or soreness. Sit in a quiet space and bring awareness to each part of your body. Starting from your toes, notice if they are curled or relaxed. Clench and unclench your leg muscles. Notice if your back is hunched over or straight. Feel whether your facial muscles are furrowed or smiling. Notice any warmth in your body or tingling sensations. Continue doing this until you feel relaxed and less stressed.

Another readily accessible mindfulness technique is mindful walking. This involves engaging all of your senses as you walk, appreciating the present moment, and noticing the sounds and smells around you. Mindful walking can be a great way to incorporate mindfulness into your daily routine without requiring a dedicated space or time. You could practice mindful walking during your lunch break, on a walk with a friend, or even while running errands.

Here is a script you can use:

Mindful walking is an opportunity to transform a simple act into a powerful exercise in presence, connecting with yourself and the world around you. You don't need to go far or walk fast. The goal is to be present with each step and each moment.

Begin by finding a comfortable walking spot, such as an outdoor area in nature, a quiet park, or a peaceful path in your home or garden.

As you stand, before taking your first step, gently bring your awareness to your body. Notice your feet on the ground. Feel the sensation of gravity pulling you gently downward, rooting you to the earth. Take a slow, deep breath in... and exhale, letting any tension begin to soften.

Now, as you begin to walk, let's bring our attention to the sensations of movement. Feel your feet making contact with the ground. Notice the subtle shift of weight from one foot to the other as you lift and place each foot. Feel the gentle roll of your foot from heel to toe. Don't try to change your pace; simply observe the natural rhythm of your steps.

Next, let's open up to the sense of sound. What can you hear around you? Perhaps the rustle of leaves, the distant hum of traffic, the chirping of birds, or the sound of your footsteps. Just notice these sounds as they arise and pass away, without judgment or attachment. Let them be part of the tapestry of your experience.

Now, gently bring your awareness to your sense of sight. Without fixing your gaze, allow your eyes to softly take in the colors, shapes, and textures around you. Notice the intricate details of a leaf, the pattern on the bark of a tree, the varying shades of green, and the way the light touches different surfaces. See if you can notice something you've never truly seen before, even in a familiar place. Simply observe, without labeling or judging.

Let's expand your awareness to your sense of smell. What scents are carried on the air? Perhaps the dampness of the earth, the sweetness of a flower, the freshness after rain, or even just the clean, open air. Take a gentle inhale and allow the aromas to fill your senses.

And finally, open to your sense of touch, beyond just your feet on the ground. Feel the air on your skin. Is it warm or cool? Notice any gentle breeze. Feel the texture of your clothing against your body. Be present with these simple, tangible sensations.

Now, bring all your senses together, allowing yourself to be fully immersed in this moment, in this walk. Feel your feet, hear the sounds, see the sights, smell the air, and feel the breeze. Every step is an opportunity to deepen your connection to the present moment, to your body, and to the world around you.

Continue walking for as long as feels comfortable, allowing each step to be a mindful step. Each moment is an opportunity for presence, for calm, and for appreciation.

Mindfulness encourages us to approach everyday experiences with curiosity, noticing things for the first time—bark on a tree to random thoughts that pop into our minds—and seeing them for what they are. One objection to practicing mindfulness is that people may not have the time to sit still in silence and engage in breath work or body scans. But you can practice mindfulness while folding laundry or washing the dishes.

While folding laundry, mindfully separate each piece of clothing, noticing the scent and if the clothes are warm. Pay attention to the creases you iron out and the texture of the fabric. Or during the dishes, notice the bubbles in the sink, the beads of water on the plate, and listen to the clinking sounds. These practices turn ordinary tasks into intentional moments of awareness.

Tai Chi

Another complementary therapy found to be beneficial for CRF is Tai chi. It is often described as a gentle, flowing exercise, almost like a moving meditation. It is rooted in traditional Chinese medicine and is a calmer form of martial arts. It combines a series of slow, deliberate movements, deep breathing, and mindfulness. Several studies have found that Tai chi can significantly reduce fatigue in cancer patients and survivors [6]. The gentle movements and deep breathing can help improve energy levels without overexerting the body, which is particularly essential for those who are already feeling depleted.

Tai chi has also been shown to improve sleep [7]. The calming, meditative aspect of Tai chi can help regulate the nervous system, promoting relaxation. Additionally, Tai chi aids in stress reduction. Its focus on mindfulness and deep breathing helps reduce stress by lowering cortisol levels and alleviating anxiety, leading to a greater sense of calm and well-being, which in turn promotes deeper, more restful sleep.

It's essential to note that when people feel exhausted, they often feel the need to rest more, and physical activity is frequently the last thing they want to do. However, this ends up being a vicious cycle because reduced physical activity and more sedentary behavior reduce energy levels even more. Tai chi is not exhausting or vigorous and is more acceptable to people struggling with fatigue. It has been found to enhance physical function by improving balance, flexibility, and muscle strength, gradually increasing physical fitness without putting excessive strain on the body.

One of the greatest strengths of Tai chi lies in its connection between mind and body. This connection can be particularly important for cancer patients, who may feel a sense of disconnect from their bodies during treatment. By focusing on gentle movements and deep breathing, Tai chi helps to cultivate a sense of body awareness and self-compassion. Essentially, Tai chi offers a gentle, holistic approach to managing CRF, addressing not just the physical symptoms but also the emotional and mental aspects.

Korean Ginseng

Korean ginseng, also known as *Panax ginseng*, has been used in traditional Chinese medicine for thousands of years, where it was once considered so valuable that it was reserved only for royalty. Ginseng was thought to "tonify Qi." Qi (pronounced "chee") is considered to be the life force that runs through our bodies. Therefore, ginseng is thought to replenish and invigorate this vital energy in the body. Ginseng is also believed to "calm the mind," which helps reduce stress and improve sleep. In Chinese medicine, herbs are thought to carry either warm or cold properties. Ginseng is classified as a warming herb, meaning it enhances blood flow and provides warmth to invigorate the body.

Scientific research supports the use of ginseng for alleviating fatigue, and one study, which included over 1,200 participants, found that individuals taking ginseng reported improved energy, encompassing both emotional and cognitive aspects [8]. Emotional energy refers to resilience against stress and depression, while cognitive energy refers to increased capacity to focus and think.

CLINICAL PEARL

A daily dose of 2,000–3,000 mg taken for two to three months has shown effectiveness in managing CRF.

Acupuncture

The sixth recommendation in the ASCO/SIO guideline is acupuncture. The potential benefits of this approach for CRF are a fascinating topic, and research in this area is still growing. In traditional Chinese medicine, acupuncture is believed to stimulate the smooth flow of Qi, the vital energy force that flows throughout the body.

Picture your body as a network of energy channels, kind of like rivers flowing through a landscape. In Chinese medicine, these channels are called meridians, and it is within these meridians that Qi flows. When you're healthy, Qi flows smoothly, maintaining balance throughout the body. However, when dealing with something like CRF, these rivers can become blocked, much like a dam stopping the flow of the river.

Acupuncture acts like a targeted dam-breaker. Chinese medicine doctors believe that acupuncture needles stimulate the flow of Qi properly. The needles help release blockages, allowing energy to flow freely.

From a Western scientific perspective, acupuncture is believed to stimulate the nervous system, triggering the release of natural chemicals in the brain, such as endorphins, serotonin, and dopamine, which are natural pain relievers and mood boosters [9]. These substances play key roles in regulating sleep, mood, and energy levels.

Though more studies are needed to fully understand the mechanisms involved, the growing body of evidence suggests that acupuncture can be a valuable tool for managing CRF. And because it's considered safe when performed by a qualified practitioner, it's often a well-tolerated therapy that patients typically find relaxing and enjoyable.

CLINICAL PEARL

My protocol for CRF is as follows: Yintang, Shenmen, PC6, HT7, CV17, CV6, ST36, SP6, KD3, LV3. I recommend twice-weekly sessions for four weeks, followed by weekly sessions for an additional four weeks. You may show this to your acupuncturist.

Yoga

Yoga originated over 5,000 years ago in ancient India. Most people are familiar with yoga and associate it with a series of postures, both standing and on the floor. There are various types of yoga, and some movements are designed for deep stretching and relaxation, while others are meant to be more physically challenging.

But there is much more to yoga than the postures. Yoga philosophy is also deeply rooted in mastering the mind through breath and meditation. It is yet another therapy that brings together body and mind.

Research consistently supports the use of yoga for reducing fatigue in cancer survivors, as it improves mood, sleep, and overall quality of life [10]. The deep breathing component of yoga promotes relaxation and helps reduce negative thought patterns, while the physical movements and postures enhance muscle health and flexibility.

Here are some yoga poses that are thought to boost energy and vitality. Start on the floor, holding each pose for two to four breaths. Remember to continue breathing deeply and slowly as you transition from one pose to another. Get creative and find a flow that you enjoy, and do the poses in any order that makes sense and feels good to you.

1. Child's Pose—Kneel on the floor, lift your arms toward the sky, and fold forward over your thighs.

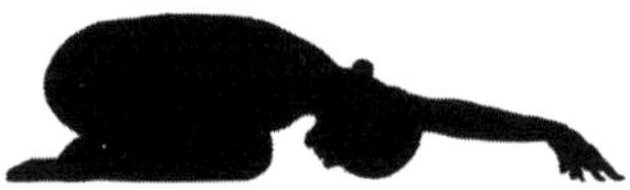

2. Cobra Pose—Transition to lie on your stomach, place your palms under your shoulders, and press up.

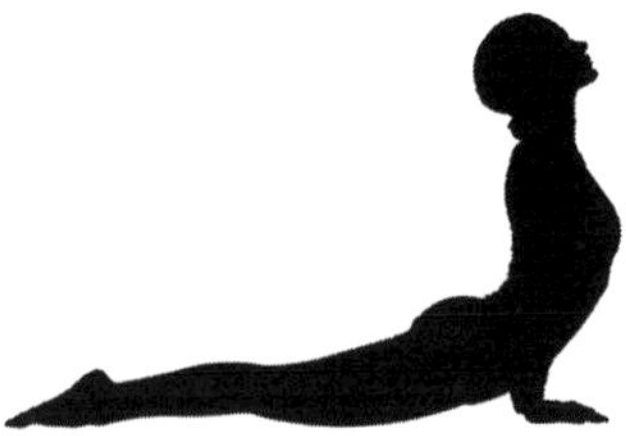

3. Camel Pose—Return to a kneeling position and gently bend backward as much as your body allows. You can look up at the sky or reach your hands toward your heels. Move only as far as feels comfortable to avoid injury.

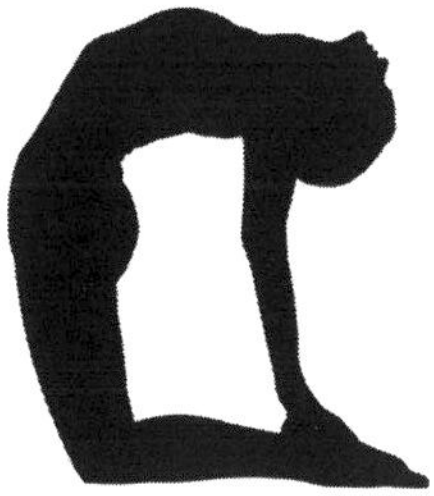

4. Bridge Pose—Lie on your back with your knees bent and feet hip-width apart. Lift your hips, clasp your hands together, and tuck your shoulder blades under you.

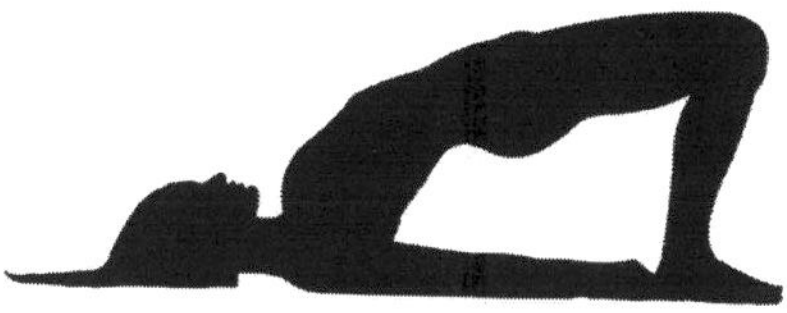

5. Downward-facing Dog—Transition to an all-fours position, lift your hips, and straighten your legs.

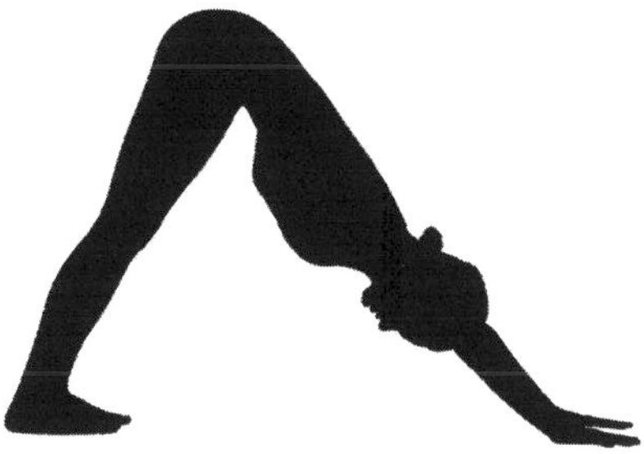

6. Chair Pose—Stand with your feet together, bend your knees, and raise your arms overhead.

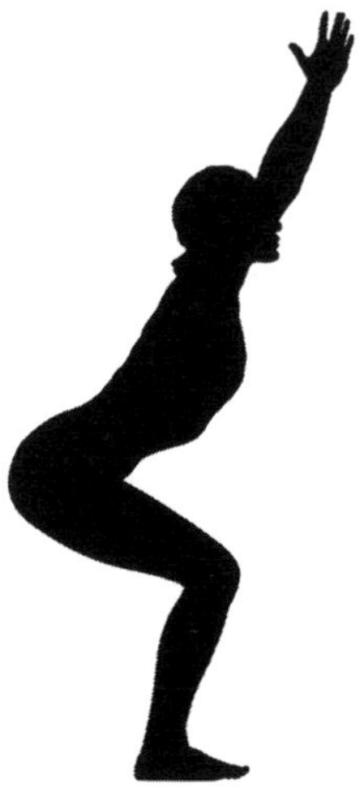

7. Tree Pose—Stand on one leg and place the sole of the opposite foot either above or below the knee, then reach your hands overhead. Remember to do both sides.

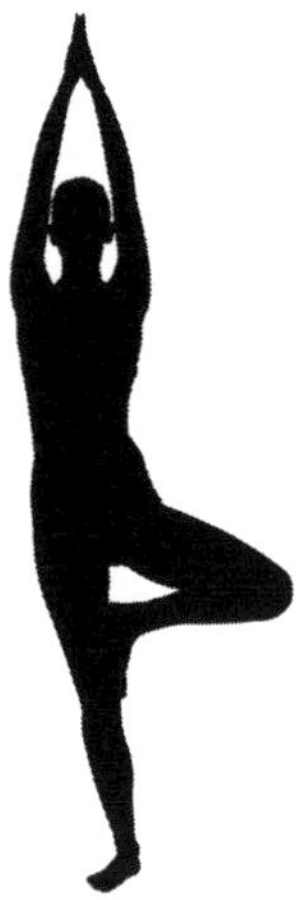

8. Warrior 1 Pose—Step forward with one leg, bend your front knee into a lunge, with your back foot turned out. Lift your arms overhead and reach up.

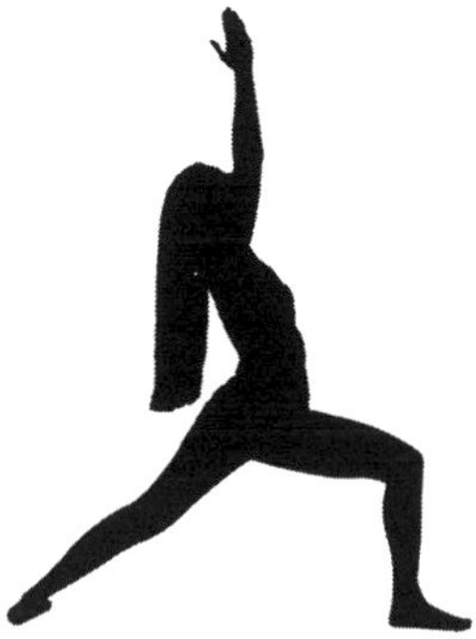

9. Warrior 2 Pose—From Warrior 1, open your hips to the side, extending your arms in front and behind. Repeat Warrior 1 and Warrior 2 on the other side.

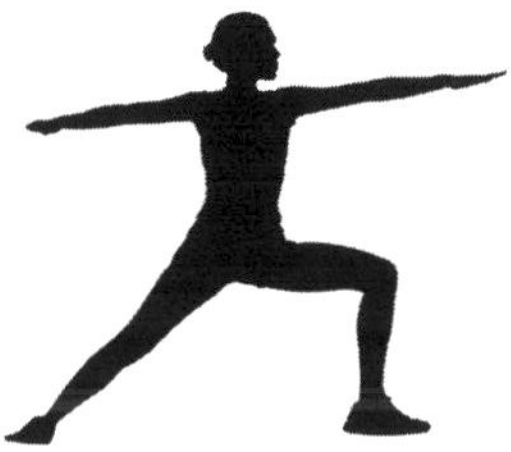

10. Mountain Pose—Stand tall with feet together, arms relaxed at your sides but engaged. Lift through the crown of your head.

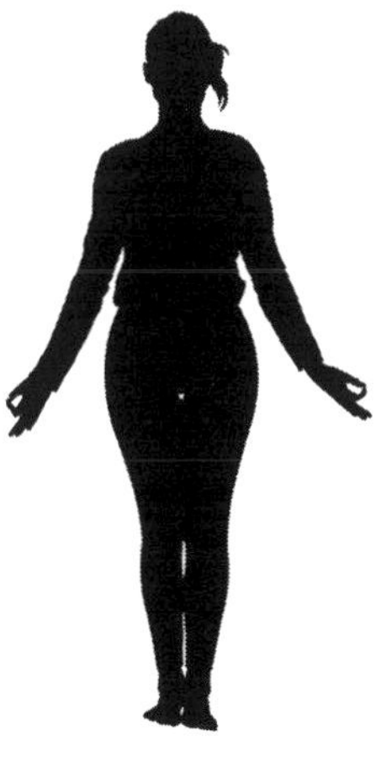

Conclusion

People experiencing long-term fatigue can become frustrated not only with feeling so exhausted but also with not knowing how to help themselves. If you feel unsure where to start, I hope this chapter has provided you with a starting point, along with some guidance and reassurance.

As mentioned earlier, you will resonate more with some ideas than others. Perhaps you enjoy yoga, but physical limitations prevent you from getting down on the floor. Tai chi might be a better fit. Or maybe you're not drawn to Chinese medicine and prefer a more vigorous workout, in which case weightlifting might be more appealing. Or perhaps you're more emotionally expressive and enjoy discussing things—CBT could be the right option for you. Alternatively, you might feel most proactive when taking medication or supplements, leading you to try ginseng.

The first step is to choose something that resonates with you and commit to it. You may have noticed that none of these recommendations involve sitting still and waiting for energy to return. Healing after cancer treatments is an active process. To boost your energy, you can't simply rest more or isolate yourself from others. You need to empower yourself to take control of your energy.

References

1 Bower JE, Lacchetti C, Alici Y, et al. Management of fatigue in adult survivors of cancer: ASCO-Society for Integrative Oncology Guideline Update. J Clin Oncol, 2024; 42(20):2456–2487.
2 Volpi E, Nazemi R, Fujita S. Muscle tissue changes with aging. Curr Open Clin Nutr Metab Care, 2004; 7:405–410.
3 Tolea MI, Galvin JE. Sarcopenia and impairment in cognitive and physical performance. Clin Interv Aging, 2015; 10:663–671.
4 Blondell SJ, Hammersley-Mather R, Veerman JL, et al. Does physical activity prevent cognitive decline and dementia? A systematic review and meta-analysis of longitudinal studies. BMC Public Health, 2014; 14:510.
5 Charade E, Baes N, Kiropoulos L. The effects of mindfulness-based interventions on symptoms of depression, anxiety and cancer related fatigue in oncology patients: a systematic review and meta-analysis. PLoS One, 2022; 17(7):e0269519.
6 Song S, Yu J, Ruan Y, et al. Ameliorative effects of Tai Chi on cancer-related fatigue: a meta-analysis of randomized controlled trials. Support Care Cancer, 2018; 26(7):2091–2102.

7 Kreutz C, Schmidt ME, Steindorf K. Effects of physical and mind-body exercise on sleep problems during and after breast cancer treatment: a systematic review and meta-analysis. Breast Cancer Res Treat, 2019; 176(1):1–15.

8 Li H, Hou T, Sun S, et al. Efficacy of ginseng oral administration and ginseng injections on cancer related fatigue: a meta-analysis. Medicine, 2022; 101:e31363.

9 Sun B, Cao X, Xin M, et al. Treatment of depression with acupuncture based on pathophysiological mechanism. Int J Gen Med, 2024; 17:347–357.

10 Hou L, Wang J, Mao M, et al. Effect of yoga on cancer-related fatigue in patients with breast cancer: a systematic review and meta-analysis. Medicine (Baltimore), 2024; 103(1):e36468.

4

The Power of Food

The food you eat can be either the safest and most powerful form of medicine or the slowest form of poison

—Ann Wigmore

This chapter is for you if:

- You eat food to survive.
- This chapter is for everyone, as nutrition is the foundation of health, and it will be one of the greatest makers or breakers of your process to improve your energy.

Imagine this: a new patient has booked a consultation. We greet each other in the waiting area, proceed into the office, and the appointment begins. The patient has recently completed grueling cancer treatments. I expect questions about how to minimize side effects or how to interpret blood work results. But the question that inevitably comes is: What should I eat?

Questions surrounding nutrition and what to eat after a cancer diagnosis are arguably top of mind for most who enter the consultation room. The information on the internet is vast, but unfortunately, it is outright confusing and contradictory. You'll read about "diets" that promise to starve cancer. Miracle foods are commonly dangled before you as the cure for your illness. Should you become a vegetarian or try fasting? Should you cut out sugar, but still eat lots of fruit? For a topic that should be so basic, food causes a lot of stress for people.

If you finish this chapter remembering anything, it should be the following sentences.

- The stress about what you eat is often worse than the food itself.
- Food and nutrition are not that complicated.

Beyond Cancer Fatigue: A Path to Reclaiming Energy, First Edition. Jessa Landmann, ND.

- Being a healthy eater is a continuum that can constantly be improved upon.
- What works for one person may not work for another.

This chapter exists to answer the question: "What should I eat?" The findings from research paint a clear picture of the nutritional landscape for those with and recovering from a cancer diagnosis. Not only are cancer survivors interested in what to eat to prevent cancer from returning, but also what to eat to have the highest energy and feel their best.

We will clear up common food myths, teach you about the most beneficial eating patterns, and explain why certain types of "fad diets" might be harmful. This chapter will teach you about a few foods to avoid and others to include in high amounts. By the end of this chapter, you will feel confident that your food choices are right for you and your body, and you will be on your way to feeling your best and living your best life.

A Note on Disordered Eating

This chapter is your guide to fueling your body for lasting, vibrant energy. This book does not promote restrictive eating patterns but trusts that you can make the best decisions for yourself. We want to support balanced, flexible eating patterns, without judgment about what choices you make, and without pressure to follow some absolute rule. This is meant to be encouragement to those who may be struggling with disordered eating.

My goal for every patient is to promote intuitive eating, which involves listening to your body. Choose foods that satisfy you and respect your hunger and fullness cues. What you feel like eating may vary from day to day, and that's okay. Not every meal or snack will be "perfect," as perfection is far from the goal. The goal is to nourish your body, enabling it to recover from cancer treatments. Avoid using the words "healthy" and "unhealthy" when thinking about what you eat day to day, and respect your changing needs, symptoms, and emotions.

The purpose of this chapter is to focus on what will give you the most energy. The guidelines provided are designed to enhance your stamina, reduce the risk of cancer recurrence, and support your recovery. It is not meant to be the moral dictator of what is the best way to eat and is certainly not meant to cause any anxiety. If this topic feels overwhelming, it's okay to take a break or seek out a qualified therapist or support group to help reassure you that your food choices are, in fact, the best for you.

Nutritional Basics

Think of your plate like an orchestra: each nutrient plays its part to create a beautiful symphony, and without a few key ingredients, the flow is not quite right. Your body needs the proper nutrients in the right amounts, and when present, our energy is optimal and flowing smoothly. A lack of essential nutrients can disrupt this balance, leading to fatigue and sluggishness. Let's start by laying the foundation for sustainable energy. Like percussion, brass, and strings, there is a powerhouse trio with nutrition. These players are proteins, carbohydrates, and fats.

Fueling Your Body: The Power of Protein

Protein is found in nearly all foods, but some are like protein superstars, packing a bigger punch than others. Getting to know who these superstars are is like unlocking the secret weapon for energy production. You may already know that protein helps build muscle, but what some people don't know is that protein is the key player in giving you the energy you need throughout the day.

Animal-based foods tend to be more concentrated sources of protein and include lean, unprocessed meats such as chicken, turkey, seafood, eggs, and dairy. If you follow a vegetarian diet, not to worry, as you can still meet your protein needs. Plant-based foods that are rich in protein include beans, lentils, chickpeas, seeds, tofu, and whole grains.

Animal-based proteins are also rich in two essential nutrients for energy: iron and vitamin B12. These are key ingredients in the production of red blood cells that carry oxygen throughout your body. Without these nutrients, you may develop anemia, which can cause the body to receive insufficient oxygen, resulting in fatigue. If you follow a vegetarian diet, you may need to supplement with iron and vitamin B12.

Here's a game-changing fact for you: people with cancer or recovering from cancer need almost double the daily protein compared to folks who haven't been through this journey. Numerous studies have highlighted a strong link between inadequate protein intake and persistent fatigue. Individuals who consume lower amounts of protein are approximately twice as likely to experience fatigue as those who consume higher amounts [1]. Even more striking, protein intake proved to be a stronger predictor of fatigue than age, insomnia, or nausea. This is a compelling argument for elevating your protein consumption.

CLINICAL PEARL

To calculate how much protein you need: If you are at a healthy weight, multiply your weight in kilograms by 1.2–1.5. If you feel you are overweight, use an online Ideal Body Weight calculator to estimate your target weight based on your sex, height, and age. Then, multiply that number in kilograms by 1.2–1.5. That number is the amount of protein in grams you need each day.

Here are some ideas to help you get the protein you need.

Food item (serving size)	Protein (in grams)	Food item (serving size)	Protein (in grams)
1 egg	6	1/2 cup beans	10
1 cup egg whites	30	1/3 cup quinoa	8
4 oz chicken	30	1/3 cup tofu	8
4 oz fish	30	1/2 cup Greek yogurt	12

Learn to Love Carbohydrates

Carbohydrates are often portrayed as the "bad guy" in nutrition, but in reality, they're your body's primary source of energy. Carbohydrates get converted into sugars, which serve as the primary fuel for our brain, organs, and muscles.

The reason for the bad reputation is that not all carbohydrates are the same. Carbohydrates generally fall into two categories: simple and complex. Simple carbs are commonly found in processed foods, white refined grains, and sugary snacks. These foods can cause "sugar crashes" and leave us feeling tired. We want to avoid these.

Complex carbs are found in foods like whole grains, vegetables, fruits, and legumes, providing a sustained energy source due to their high fiber, vitamin, and mineral content, which also helps enhance our energy levels. It is the complex carbs that we should focus on.

Fruits and vegetables are essential components of the carbohydrate family. These foods have natural colors, and foods with color are rich in antioxidants. Antioxidants are directly responsible for lowering inflammation. Inflammation, as you now understand, is a significant contributor to fatigue. Research indicates that when people load their plates with an abundance of fruits and vegetables, inflammation decreases and energy levels improve [2].

Aim for at least five to six servings of fruits and vegetables each day. Think of it as eating the rainbow!

Food item	Serving size	Food item	Serving size
Blueberries	1/2 to 1 cup	Carrots	12 baby or 1 whole
Kiwi	2 whole fruits	Spinach and other greens	1/2 cup cooked or 2 cups raw
Grapes	15–20 pieces	Bell pepper	1 whole piece
Melon	1/2 to 1 cup	Broccoli or cauliflower	1/2 cup
Strawberries	8 pieces	Sweet potato	1/2 cup mashed
Banana, apple, orange, grapefruit, peach, pear	1 whole fruit	Green beans	1/2 cup

The Truth About Fats: Your Energy Ally

Fats, like carbs, have also been misunderstood and unfairly demonized. But not all fats are the same. Fats are divided into two forms: saturated and unsaturated. Saturated fats are typically solids, such as those found around the edges of meats and in butter. Unsaturated fats are typically liquids, such as those found in oily fish and olive oil. Picture saturated fats as the ones that are thick and clog arteries, while liquids are slippery and allow blood to flow smoothly.

Your focus should be on consuming enough of the unsaturated, healthy fats found in foods like creamy avocados, nuts, seeds, oily fish, and olive oil. These foods are rich in omega-3 fatty acids, often referred to as the "good fats," and help lower inflammation in the body. Studies have shown that consuming foods rich in these beneficial fats can improve people's energy levels [3].

Aim for at least two to three servings of healthy fats per day.

Food item	Serving size	Food item	Serving size
Olive oil	1 tsp	Avocado	1/2 whole fruit
Nuts (almond, cashew)	Small handful	Fish	Size of palm of hand
Nut butters	1.5 tbsp	Seeds (chia, pumpkin)	1.5 tbsp

REFLECTION POINT

Begin to be curious about what you are eating. Make sure you calculate your protein needs before proceeding. Reflect on what you have eaten in the past few days. Have you consumed five to six servings of fruits and vegetables and two to three servings of fats? Do you tend to eat a lot of simple carbs or complex carbs?

And regarding fats, do you consume more saturated or unsaturated fats? If you're a vegetarian, have you been supplementing with iron and vitamin B12? Consider keeping a food diary if you haven't done so before.

Beyond the Basics—What to Eat After a Cancer Diagnosis to Combat Cancer-related Fatigue and Reduce Your Risk of a Recurrence

The main goal of this book is to help you reduce cancer-related fatigue. As a bonus, the nutritional strategies discussed also help to fight cancer and reduce your risk of a recurrence. Eating nutritious food isn't just about nourishing your body and improving your energy—it supports your strength, your resilience, and your long-term vitality. The saying "you are what you eat" resonates deeply here. This couldn't be more true. The choices we make with food have a tangible effect on how our bodies function, for better or worse.

Unfortunately, many cancer patients receive little to no nutritional advice. As a cancer survivor reading this book, know that the insights and suggestions here are not just hopeful ideas—they are grounded in extensive research and designed to be fundamental to your care and well-being.

The Good, The Bad, The Ugly

Let's talk about what types of foods people with cancer should eat and what types they should avoid. When it comes to nutritional advice, the research is clear.

The "Goods"

When it comes to high energy levels, cancer prevention, and overall good health, the most potent nutrients are found in fruits, vegetables, high-fiber foods, and healthy fats.

Fruits and vegetables are rich in pigments of red, orange, yellow, and green. Think berries, citrus, tomatoes, bell peppers, sweet potatoes, and leafy greens. As mentioned earlier, these colors provide a rich source of antioxidants that lower inflammation and improve energy. High fruit and vegetable intake not only enhances energy in cancer survivors [4], but it is also helpful for other chronic fatigue syndromes [5].

High fruit and vegetable intake is associated with better cancer outcomes, including a lower risk of recurrence and improved overall survival. One study found that men with prostate cancer who consumed the highest amount of fruits and vegetables had a 53% lower risk of cancer recurrence [6]. This has also been found in survivors of breast cancer and colon cancer [7].

Next up is fiber, which is found in fruits, vegetables, beans, cereal fibers (such as bran and oats), and other whole grains, including wheat, rice, barley, and quinoa. Dietary fiber is considered one of the powerhouses of foods, as it has been found to reduce the risk of type 2 diabetes, cardiovascular disease, and cancer [8]. The reasons for this are that the nutrients found in fiber lower inflammation, lower blood sugar levels, improve the immune system, and enhance the gut microbiome. High-fiber foods not only improve energy [9], but are also linked to a lower risk of breast cancer, colon cancer, stomach cancer, and possibly even brain cancer [10].

Finally, healthy fats round out our discussion of the "goods." As discussed earlier, these include foods such as avocado, nuts, seeds, fish, and olive oil. Healthy fats are anti-inflammatory and beneficial for all cells in the body, including the heart and brain.

Most research on the benefits of omega-3 fats for cancer is found in studies on the Mediterranean diet (MedDiet). The MedDiet is associated with better energy levels [3] and lower rates of cancer recurrence. We will discuss the MedDiet in more detail in the next section.

CLINICAL PEARL

For a moment, let's return to that situation where the patient is in the consultation room and asks that inevitable question: What should I eat? The first step is to ensure you are getting all the necessary nutrients—five to six servings of fruits and vegetables, high fiber from whole grains, and two to three servings of healthy fats each day. The second step is to meet your required protein needs. This is the minimum you should aim for each day.

The "Bads"

So far, we've covered foods that are helpful in boosting energy and preventing cancer recurrence. However, it's just as important to understand which foods may be best to avoid, as they lower energy and are also linked to adverse cancer outcomes. These foods include red meat, processed meats, excessive sugar from processed foods and sweets, and alcohol.

Red meat includes beef, pork, goat, and lamb and is linked with an increased risk of cancer [11], namely cancers of the digestive system, such as colon cancer, esophageal cancer, stomach cancer, liver cancer, and pancreatic cancer. For cancer survivors, high red meat intake is linked with an increased risk of recurrence in breast cancer, colon cancer, prostate cancer, and digestive cancers [12]. It is best to limit red meat consumption to once per week.

In contrast, white meat refers to chicken and turkey, and there appears to be a much lower risk associated with consuming these animal products. Therefore, if you are a meat-eater or are trying to ensure you meet your daily protein requirements, these meats can be consumed without much concern.

We also have processed meats, such as hot dogs, cold cuts, ham, bacon, and sausages. Processed meats are strongly linked to the development of cancer, so the recommendation is to avoid them altogether [13].

High sugar intake is next to be discussed. You may have heard that sugar "feeds" cancer and that cutting it completely will be the answer. While it's more complex than that, being smart about the types of sugar we eat can make a difference in how we feel.

Where people get confused is the type of sugar they should avoid. The sugar to avoid is *added sugar* found in soda, sweet syrups in coffee drinks, the piles of sugar in baked goods, and the added sugar that is often hidden in items like prepackaged sauces, granola bars, and other canned goods. These are the sugars to avoid. This does not include natural sugars found in fruits and vegetables. We should limit processed foods and sweets to once per week.

Finally, let's discuss alcohol. Like cigarettes and processed meats, alcohol is known to cause cancer in humans. There is no safe level of alcohol consumption when it comes to cancer risk, and the general recommendation is to avoid it altogether.

It's essential to know the truth about alcohol and our energy: it steals it. It raises our blood sugar, contributes to muscle loss, and disrupts our sleep. Alcohol can also disrupt our natural circadian rhythm, interfering with the production of melatonin [14].

CLINICAL PEARL

When choosing your foods, remember these two words: sufficient and consistent. Ask yourself, concerning the goods and the bads: "Are you getting a sufficient amount of the good (fruits, vegetables, fibers, healthy fats) consistently, while avoiding the bads as much as possible?" If your answer is yes, then you should feel confident that you are doing a good job.

The Ugly

There is a noticeable trend in the cancer population about attitudes toward food. It is not uncommon to hear patients express the idea that they caused their cancer by eating "too many cookies." The advice on the internet about what to eat is completely contradictory and confusing. My patients have heard me say many times that the stress about what you are eating is likely worse than what you are actually eating.

Cancer survivors may also get advice about nutrition from well-meaning friends or support groups. They have heard the story of someone's friend who cut out dairy, meat, sugar, and wheat and beat cancer. People may start to label foods as "healthy" and "unhealthy" and become restrictive about their eating patterns or fearful of what they are eating.

However, it is strongly discouraged to label foods as healthy and unhealthy, as it can create anxiety. This kind of labeling can lead to obsessive restriction about food and does not serve your well-being. The reason this book dedicates significant space to the topic of nutrition is to help you address these negative emotions and to help you feel like an expert on the subject of food.

When it comes to the "ugly," this refers to the overly restrictive ways of eating for fear of being responsible for your cancer. It is ugly to feel shame about eating something that you read on the internet is bad for you or something a well-meaning friend told you not to eat. The anxiety surrounding food will also not help with energy levels.

Orthorexia is not an official eating disorder, but it's a recognized form of disordered eating. It involves an unhealthy, obsessive, and extreme fixation on consuming only "pure" and "healthy" foods, primarily focusing on the quality and cleanliness of the diet [15]. It often involves rigid rules about what one eats, including the avoidance of entire food groups. However, disordered eating can lead to severe nutritional deficiencies, possibly endangering someone's health, and is linked with depression and anxiety [16].

There is evidence of orthorexic behaviors, particularly in women with breast cancer [17]. Restrictive and altered food habits are associated with weight loss and possibly malnutrition, even when there is no intention to lose weight. Weight loss can be risky for some people with cancer, especially when one considers that 20% of cancer patients die from malnutrition [18].

In one small study of women with breast cancer, the researchers found that 44% changed their eating habits after their diagnosis and that orthorexia was linked to fear of recurrence and higher internet use [19]. The well-meaning "wellness warriors" of the internet preach about "the best way to eat," and so if you feel you often get sucked into the online rhetoric about healthy eating, avoiding these websites will be helpful for you.

This rising trend should necessitate the development of clear guidelines surrounding nutrition advice for cancer survivors. Policymakers and educators should understand how misinformation can lead to disordered eating and strive to promote healthy relationships with food, focusing on the foods that contribute to strength, improved immune function, better sleep, increased energy, and a reduced risk of recurrence.

We need to strike a balance between informed nutritional choices and avoiding extreme dietary restrictions. Nutrition for cancer is not that complicated, as this book will continually strive to emphasize. You don't need to avoid entire food groups, and you don't need to be perfect. Focus on enjoying fruits, vegetables, fiber, healthy fats, and lean, unprocessed meats, while being mindful of red meat, processed foods, and alcohol. That's the core of it. Support your energy with knowledge and kindness, and nurture it without unnecessary stress. Food should be an ally in healing, not your enemy.

For Healthcare Practitioners

Women with breast cancer may be more susceptible to developing orthorexia, and therefore, diligent screening should take place among this population [20]. One validated screening tool that can help is the ORTO-R, which is available in both a 6-item short form and a more comprehensive 15-item expanded version [21].

This bears repeating: healthcare professionals, policymakers, and educators must be well-versed in the nuances of nutrition for cancer survivors. Providing confident advice on the best foods to support healing, promote well-being, and minimize the recurrence of illness is paramount. The focus should be on nourishment and abundance, not restrictive diets that could inadvertently lead to malnourishment and hinder recovery. Given the concerning prevalence of disordered eating, particularly among women with a history of cancer, promoting a healthy and balanced relationship with food must be part of comprehensive cancer care.

Beyond the Basics: Fad Diets

A fad diet is a recommended way of eating for a particular health condition that promises to be the cure or have an impactful way of influencing the course of that health condition. Fad diets often strongly recommend specific foods to eat and those to avoid. In some cases, they can be restrictive and potentially harm your health and energy levels. These fad diets often tie into orthorexic thoughts.

Here's where it gets interesting, though. There may be certain situations in which a fad diet could be potentially helpful. Fad diets are sometimes referred to as therapeutic diets. A therapeutic diet refers to a prescribed meal plan tailored to an individual to improve their health, manage symptoms, and support recovery.

The difference between a fad diet and a therapeutic diet is that the latter is explicitly tailored to you and your situation, will not cause you harm, and has research supporting its use. A fad diet may recommend a particular way of eating for *all* people, is not personalized, does not have substantial research for a specific condition, and may be risky or harmful to you.

Below are the six most commonly asked about diets in clinical practice. We'll examine their pros and cons through the lens of nourishing your body to enhance your energy and support long-term recovery.

Fad Diet 1: Mediterranean Diet

The MedDiet is an approved therapeutic diet and is the top contender for people recovering from cancer who want to get their energy back. The MedDiet is rich in fruits, vegetables, whole grains, nuts, seeds, and legumes and allows moderate amounts of animal protein (from fish, white meat, and dairy). It avoids red meat, refined grains, and processed foods. It's sometimes referred to as a plant-based diet because it prioritizes plant foods but allows for some animal protein.

The MedDiet can boost your energy in several ways. It reduces inflammation, improves sleep [22], and lessens the symptoms of depression [23]. This style of eating is high in fiber, antioxidants, and healthy fats, which is what we strive for. Additionally, the MedDiet is widely accepted by people because it is flexible, non-restrictive and is more about enjoying flavorful food than giving things up.

Many people in my practice ask about what types of foods they should eat to prevent a cancer recurrence. Several extensive studies have shown that people who stick to a MedDiet style of eating pattern have a 10–20% reduced risk of cancer recurrence [24]. That's a powerful reason to pay attention.

Because the MedDiet has the fewest restrictions, is delicious and enjoyable, and offers numerous health benefits, it is one of the most sustainable ways of eating for someone navigating life with or after cancer, supporting both your energy and your long-term well-being.

Fad Diet 2: Time-restricted Eating

Time-restricted eating (TRE) involves alternating periods of eating and fasting on a consistent schedule. The focus is more on *when* you eat rather than *what* you eat.

The most typical pattern is an 8- to 10-hour eating window, with the rest of the day spent drinking water or tea.

One fascinating aspect of TRE is how it helps our bodies restore a natural circadian rhythm. The circadian rhythm is our body's internal 24-hour clock that responds specifically to external signals such as food and light exposure. It regulates our hormones, appetite, digestion, body temperature, and sleep. When the timing of our meals aligns with this rhythm, our health improves, often leading to better energy and sleep.

Studies on TRE for reducing fatigue have shown encouraging results. It has been found that not only does TRE improve energy, but it also helps eliminate excess weight and improve mood [25]. It is not meant to be a calorie-reduction plan, but by default, fewer calories may be consumed. One study specifically on women with breast cancer found that it may be associated with lower recurrence rates [26].

One reason TRE is so well-received is that it does not restrict what you eat, but only limits the time you have to eat. There's little downside to trying TRE, and it's considered a safe and approved therapeutic diet.

Case Study

Alice is a breast cancer survivor. She was diagnosed with stage III breast cancer and underwent surgery, radiation, and chemotherapy for her treatment. She came to see me when she was two months posttreatment. Her primary reason for seeing me was extreme fatigue, poor sleep, and constipation.

She was a busy mother of three. Her days were spent working as an accountant, and her evenings were spent driving her children to their competitive sports. She admitted she did not eat breakfast, but would have time for lunch. Dinners were often late at night after everyone got home from their activities and were often the largest meal of the day.

I explained how the circadian rhythm works and that the body prefers to have a large meal in the morning when metabolism and digestion are at their optimal levels. Additionally, I mentioned that the size of meals should be at its lowest in the evening, when digestion slows down. Having a large meal at night may be impacting her sleep and contributing to constipation. I convinced her to start eating breakfast as the main meal of the day and to eat dinner early, before she started driving the children to their sports activities. I also instructed her specifically to only eat between the hours of 9 am and 6 pm.

She noticed within two weeks that her energy had improved from a 5/10 to an 8/10, she was sleeping through the night, and she was experiencing daily bowel movements.

Fad Diet 3: Ketogenic Diet

When it comes to cancer recovery and specifically tackling cancer-related fatigue, the current research on ketogenic diets is limited. However, we can rely on clinical experience and nutritional common sense to assess whether the ketogenic diet might be beneficial.

The traditional ketogenic diet is very high in fat (often including red meat, bacon, and butter), with minimal intake of carbohydrates, like fruits, vegetables, and grains. Right away, we can see that this does not align with what we've learned so far about fueling your body optimally.

Recently, some "keto-like" diets have been recommended. They emphasize healthy fats (excluding red meat, bacon, and butter), allow more fruits, vegetables, and whole grains, and encourage higher protein intake from oily fish and lean white meat. These diets resemble the MedDiet, offering healthy fats, fiber, fruits, vegetables, and balanced protein. Any energy benefits would likely be similar to those of the MedDiet.

Currently, a *traditional* ketogenic diet isn't recommended for improving energy and aiding recovery from cancer-related fatigue. The focus on very high fat and very low intake of fruits, vegetables, and protein doesn't match the nutritional needs of cancer survivors. However, if you're considering a modified "keto-like" approach, it may offer energy-boosting benefits comparable to the MedDiet, better supporting overall health and well-being.

Fad Diet 4: Paleolithic Diets (Paleo)

The paleo diet, also known as the ancestral or Stone Age diet, is based on the concept of eating like our hunter-gatherer ancestors did. It focuses on whole foods such as fruits, vegetables, nuts, seeds, and fish. The advantages of this eating pattern include its high content of antioxidants and healthy fats, which help reduce inflammation. It may lower inflammation to a similar degree as the MedDiet and can also help boost energy levels [27].

However, the paleo diet restricts some foods that are beneficial for our health, especially when it comes to cancer. Grains and legumes are discouraged because humans didn't evolve with them. However, as you've learned, grains and legumes are rich sources of fiber, which benefits the microbiome.

Legume consumption may also be associated with lower rates of cancer. People who eat a higher amount of legumes may have a lower risk of colon cancer [28] and endometrial cancer [29]. Additionally, grains and legumes are beneficial for managing blood sugar, lowering cholesterol, and may help with weight management. Higher fiber intake has been linked to a lower risk of cancer recurrence. It seems there isn't a strong reason to limit these foods from our daily diet.

Therefore, this is one example of a fad diet that is unlikely to be strongly recommended. The paleo diet may offer some benefits, such as being anti-inflammatory and helping reduce fatigue, but it may not be beneficial for overall cancer wellness. It's another example of a diet trend that cancer survivors should weigh out the pros and cons.

Fad Diet 5: Vegetarian Diets

Vegetarian diets exclude meat, such as chicken, turkey, pork, and beef, but some include limited animal products, including fish, dairy, and eggs. These diets focus on plant-based foods, including fruits, vegetables, grains, legumes, nuts, and seeds, which are rich in antioxidants and have anti-inflammatory properties. People who choose vegetarian diets are often health-conscious and engage in energy-supporting behaviors, such as regular exercise [30]. Vegetarian diets are also associated with a lower risk of cardiovascular disease [31].

However, this approach may not be suitable for everyone. Generally, you need to eat a larger volume of food to get the protein you need. For people with cancer who have a higher requirement for protein, this can be challenging if other factors affect food intake, such as lack of appetite or nausea.

Because vegetarian diets may cause protein deficiency, these eating patterns could be too restrictive and risky for anyone who has lost weight, is underweight, has issues with bone density, or is elderly. Protein is the key building block for muscle and bone, and as we will discuss in Chapter 10, losing muscle can be dangerous.

Since vegetarian diets contain less animal protein, they can also be lower in specific key vitamins and minerals that are primarily found in animal products, such as iron, vitamin B12, and calcium. Low iron and vitamin B12 levels can lead to anemia, which can cause people to feel drained and weak.

When it comes to fatigue specifically, due to the lack of animal protein, this may not be the most supportive way of eating. There can be a proper time and place for vegetarian dietary patterns, but unless you can consume a large quantity of plant-based foods to meet your protein needs, this approach may not be the most effective way to address fatigue.

Fad Diet 6: Juicing

Among popular fad diets, juicing tends to offer the fewest overall benefits for sustained energy and long-term well-being. While it's true that juicing increases your intake of fruits and vegetables, and it can help with hydration, that's about it. Juices are very high in sugar, and they can lead to unwanted spikes in blood sugar levels. The other downsides of relying heavily on juicing are that it almost completely strips away two crucial food components of energy: fiber and protein.

There may be times when a small amount of fresh-pressed fruit or vegetable juice could be beneficial, such as when someone has a low appetite or is experiencing difficulty swallowing. However, long juice fasts are generally discouraged and can be detrimental to your overall energy.

Conclusion

As you navigate your recovery and work toward regaining energy, the recurring theme is balanced and informed choices. Some dietary approaches, like the MedDiet and mindful TRE, emerge as strong allies in boosting energy and supporting long-term health; others, like prolonged juicing, may not offer the well-rounded nourishment needed and could even be counterproductive.

The foundation of a nourishing, energizing diet includes an abundance of fruits and vegetables, wholesome fiber, healthy fats, with adequate lean protein. It's about finding balance between real, satisfying foods while being mindful of excess red and processed meat, added sugars and alcohol. More than anything, it's about fostering a peaceful, informed and confident relationship with food, free from guilt and restrictive extremes. When you eat with awareness and compassion, food stops being something that limits you and instead becomes a powerful force that restores and uplifts your life and energy.

References

1 Prado CM, Lieffers JR, McCargar LJ, et al. Prevalence and clinical implications of sarcopenic obesity in patients with solid tumours of the respiratory and gastrointestinal tracts: a population-based study. Lancet Oncol, 2008; 9:629–635.
2 Zick SM, Colacino J, Cornellier M, et al. Fatigue reduction diet in breast cancer survivors: a pilot randomized clinical trial. Breast Cancer Res Treat, 2016; 161(2):299–310.
3 Alfano CM, Imayama I, Neuhouser ML, et al. Fatigue, inflammation and omega-3 and omega-6 fatty acid intake among breast cancer survivors. J Clin Oncol, 2012; 30(12):1280–1287.
4 Kleckner AS, Kleckner IR, Renn CL, et al. Dietary composition, meal timing, and cancer-related fatigue: insights from women's healthy eating and living study. Cancer Nurs, 2025; 48(1):19–30.
5 Hasse U, Herpich C, Norman K. Anti-inflammatory diets and fatigue. Nutrients, 2019; 11(10):2315.

6 Liu VN, Van Blarigan EL, Zhang L, et al. Associations between plant-based diets and risk of disease progression in men with prostate cancer. JAMA Netw Open, 2024; 7(5):e249053.

7 Parohan M, Anjom-Shoae J, Nasiri M, et al. Dietary total antioxidant capacity and mortality from all causes, cardiovascular and cancer: a systematic review and dose-response meta-analysis of prospective cohort studies. Eur J Nutr, 2019; 48(6):2175–2189.

8 Kabisch S, Hajir J, Sukhobaevsaia V, et al. Impact of dietary fibre on inflammation in humans. Int J Mol Sci, 2025; 26(5):2000.

9 Kenkhuis MF, van Dujnhoven FJB, van Roekel EH, et al. Longitudinal associations of fibre, vegetables, fruit intake with quality of life and fatigue in colorectal cancer survivors up to 24 months post treatment. Am J Clin Nutr, 2022; 115(3):822–832.

10 Saadh MJ, Alleia OQB, Kareem RA, et al. From gut to brain: the impact of short-chain fatty acids on brain cancer. Neuromolecular Med, 2025; 27(1):10.

11 Lunn JC, Kuhnle G, Mai V, et al. The effect of heme in red and processed meat on the endogenous formation of N-nitroso compounds in the upper gastrointestinal tract. Carcinogenesis, 2007; 28:685–690.

12 Sivasubramanian BP, Dave M, Panchal V, et al. Comprehensive review of red meat consumption and the risk of cancer. Cureus, 2023; 15(9):e45324.

13 Farvid MS, Sidahmed E, Spence ND, et al. Consumption of red meat and processed meat and cancer incidence: a systematic review and meta-analysis of prospective studies. Eur J Epidemiol, 2021; 36(9):937–951.

14 Meyrel M, Rolland B, Geoffroy PA. Alterations in circadian rhythms following alcohol use: a systematic review. Prog Neuropsychopharmacol Biol Psych, 2020; 99:109831.

15 Saraswati P, Nagendraswamy C. Orthorexia nervosa – a review. Int J Psychiatry Nurs, 2015; 1:64–67.

16 Sander J, Moessner M, Bauer S. Depression, anxiety and eating disorder related impairment: moderators in female adolescents and young adults. Int J Environ Res Public Health, 2021; 18:2779.

17 Aslan H, Aktürk Ü. Demographic characteristics, nutritional behaviors, and orthorexic tendencies of women with breast cancer: a case-control study. Eat Weight Disord, 2020; 25:1365–1375.

18 Gebremedhin TK, Cherie A, Tolera BD, et al. Prevalence and risk factors of malnutrition among adult cancer patients receiving chemotherapy treatment in cancer center: a cross-sectional study. Heliyon, 2021; 7:e07362.

19 Waterman M, Lee RM, Carter JC, et al. Orthorexia symptoms and disordered eating behaviours in young women with cancer. Eat Behav, 2022; 47:101672.

20 Zoghbi R, Awad E, Matta C, et al. Prevalence of orthorexic tendencies and their correlates among Lebanese patients with cancer. Percept Mot Skills, 2023; 130(5):1952–1969.

21 Barrada JR, Roncero M. Bidimensional structure of the orthorexia: development and initial validation of a new instrument. Ann Psychol, 2018; 34(2):283–291.

22 Patel A, Cheung J. The effect of a mediterranean diet and chrononutrition on sleep quality: a scoping review. Nutr J, 2025; 24:31.

23 Yin W, Löf M, Chen R, et al. Mediterranean diet and depression: a population-based cohort study. Int J Behav Nutr Phys, 2021; 18:153.

24 Molina-Montes E, Salamanca-Fernandez E, Garcia-Villanova B, et al. The impact of plant-based dietary patterns on cancer-related outcomes: a rapid review and meta-analysis. Nutrients, 2020; 12(7):2010.

25 O'Donnell E, Shapiro Y, Comander A, et al. Pilot study to assess prolonged overnight fasting in breast cancer survivors (longfast). Breast Cancer Res Treat, 2022; 193(3):579–587.

26 Marinac CR, Nelson SH, Breen CI, et al. Prolonged nightly fasting and breast cancer. JAMA Oncol, 2016; 2(8):1049–1055.

27 Whalen KA, McCullough ML, Flanders WD, et al. Paleolithic and mediterranean diet pattern scores are inversely associated with biomarkers of inflammation and oxidative balance in adults. J Nutr, 2016; 146(6):1217–1226.

28 Jin S, Je Y. Nuts and legumes consumption and risk of colorectal cancer: a systematic review and meta-analysis. Eur J Epidemiol, 2022; 37(6):569–585.

29 Zhong XS, Ge J, Chen SW, et al. Association between dietary isoflavones in soy and legumes and endometrial cancer. J Acad Nutr Diet, 2018; 118(4):637–651.

30 Puentes DMQ, Ortega MS, Ruiz-Mamani PG, et al. Nutritional knowledge, physical activity, mood, body satisfaction, and life satisfaction in vegetarians and nonvegetarians. J Nutr Metab, 2025; 2025:1907455.

31 Landry MJ, Senkus KE, Mangels AR, et al. Vegetarian dietary patterns and cardiovascular risk factors and disease prevention: An umbrella review of systematic reviews. Am J Prev Cardiol. 2024; 20:100868.

Part II

How Hormones Contribute to Cancer-related Fatigue

5

Thyroid Health: Your Energy Engine

> *The higher your energy level, the more efficient your body. The more efficient your body, the better you feel, and the more you will use your talent to produce outstanding results*
>
> —Tony Robbins

This chapter is especially relevant if you have experienced any of the following:

- Radiation treatment involving the head, neck, upper chest, or spine.
- Total body irradiation before a stem cell transplant.
- Use of tyrosine kinase inhibitors (e.g., Lenvatinib, Sunitinib, Sorafenib, Imatinib, Nilotinib, Axitinib).
- Use of immune checkpoint inhibitors (e.g., Pembrolizumab, Atezolizumab, Ipilimumab, Nivolumab).
- Partial or complete removal of the thyroid gland.
- Treatment for thyroid cancer with radioactive iodine (I-131).

Hormones play an intricate role in our overall well-being, especially when it comes to energy, mood, and sleep. A crucial player in hormone health is the thyroid gland, a small yet powerful organ situated in the neck. Its main job is to produce thyroid hormones, T4 and T3, that influence nearly every cell and organ in the body. Disruptions to thyroid function, whether resulting in underactivity (hypothyroidism) or overactivity (hyperthyroidism), can significantly contribute to cancer-related fatigue, adding another layer of complexity to this already complicated condition.

Beyond Cancer Fatigue: A Path to Reclaiming Energy, First Edition. Jessa Landmann, ND.

Think of your thyroid as the captain of your body's energy ship. Thyroid hormones give energy to all of the tissues in our body. These hormones are key regulators of energy production, body temperature, digestion, growth, heart, and nerve function. When thyroid hormone levels are low, as in hypothyroidism, many systems slow down. You may experience symptoms such as coldness, constipation, irregular menstrual cycles, dry skin, brittle nails, hair loss, brain fog, low mood, or unexplained weight gain. Given all these symptoms, it is understandable how people would feel profound fatigue.

Hyperthyroidism, on the other hand, occurs when the thyroid gland produces excessive amounts of hormone. While it might seem counterintuitive that an overactive thyroid could lead to fatigue, this is undoubtedly the case. The overproduction of thyroid hormones results in too much energy in the body, leading to weight loss, increased heart rate, nervousness and anxiety, sleep disturbance, sweating, diarrhea, ironically, and extreme fatigue.

Both hypo- and hyperthyroidism can dramatically impact an individual's quality of life. The relentless fatigue tied to thyroid dysfunction often leads to reduced activity, muscle weakness, difficulty concentrating, memory issues, and low mood.

People with a history of cancer, especially those with a history of specific treatment regimens, as we'll discuss shortly, should be aware of the heightened risk of thyroid dysfunction and ask proactively to have blood work completed if it has not been routinely screened for in the past. We'll outline recommended blood tests for thyroid function at the end of this chapter. Let's explore how cancer can affect the thyroid and, most importantly, what you can do to start feeling better.

Thyroid Cancer

Thyroid cancer is the ninth most commonly diagnosed malignancy worldwide. Rates have steadily increased over the years, and the condition affects more women than men. It may initially present as a lump in the throat and is typically diagnosed after routine imaging, such as ultrasounds, and potentially a biopsy. If the tumor is localized, full or ideally partial removal of the thyroid gland is performed.

If the entire thyroid is removed, you'll require lifelong T4 therapy since the thyroid is the only part of the body that produces thyroid hormones. However, even with prescribed T4 medication, many individuals still experience side effects, with fatigue being a common struggle. In one study, the prevalence of long-term fatigue in thyroid cancer survivors was 42% [1].

There is evidence that T4 replacement therapy, on its own, does not significantly increase thyroid hormone levels and also does not alleviate symptoms in many individuals [2]. That's why some people might benefit from additional approaches to better support thyroid function, strategies we'll examine later in this chapter.

Breast Cancer

If you're a breast cancer survivor, your risk of developing hypothyroidism is higher than average. There are already many reasons survivors of breast cancer will struggle with fatigue, and so adding one more thing to the mix is a tough pill to swallow.

A major Danish study published in 2020 tracked 44,574 breast cancer survivors over an average of 8.4 years after their diagnosis and treatment [3]. The results of this robust trial indicate that women with a history of breast cancer have a higher likelihood of thyroid dysfunction than women without a history of breast cancer. The risk was especially high in women who underwent both radiation and chemotherapy.

Women who are prescribed Tamoxifen have also been found to experience a mild and transient hypothyroidism within the first year of treatment [4]. Tamoxifen is an estrogen-blocking medication commonly used to treat estrogen-positive breast cancers. Given that about 75% of all breast cancers are estrogen-positive, this is a large population of women who should be routinely screened for thyroid dysfunction.

If you're a breast cancer survivor struggling with ongoing fatigue, it's worth talking to your doctor about your thyroid. You'll find recommended blood tests at the end of this chapter, along with practical steps to support your thyroid and help you feel more like yourself again. You deserve to have the best quality of life after going through so much already.

Immunotherapy-associated Thyroid Dysfunction

Immunotherapy has been one of the most significant breakthroughs in cancer treatment and has become a key part of treatment protocols for many different tumor types. Two commonly prescribed types are immune checkpoint inhibitors (ICIs) and tyrosine kinase inhibitors (TKIs). These medications are not without side effects and can cause inflammation in nearly any organ, with the thyroid gland being especially vulnerable.

These drugs can cause inflammation of the thyroid, which might lead to a permanently underactive thyroid and necessitate long-term T4 replacement [5]. The prevalence of thyroid dysfunction in patients treated with these drugs ranges from 10% [6] to 50% [7]. Sometimes doctors use a combination of immunotherapy drugs, making it even more likely that the thyroid will be affected [8].

Detecting thyroid problems early benefits your long-term health. If you're on immunotherapy and feel constantly fatigued, discuss this with your healthcare team, as it may be an important factor not to be missed.

Head and Neck Cancer

Head and neck cancers include tumors that originate anywhere from the neck upwards, excluding the brain. They may occur in the salivary glands, voice box, tongue, lips, throat, or nose. These cancers are commonly treated with radiation, and because the thyroid gland is located in the neck near the radiation field, it is often affected.

The risk of developing hypothyroidism after treatment is significant. Approximately 40–50% of people who have been treated for head and neck cancers go on to develop hypothyroidism [9]. This typically requires long-term T4 therapy, highlighting another group of patients who need careful thyroid monitoring.

Hashimoto's Thyroiditis

Thyroid issues may already be present before a cancer diagnosis, and one of the most common causes of hypothyroidism is an autoimmune condition called Hashimoto's. Autoimmune diseases happen when the body's immune system mistakenly targets its own organs as foreign invaders, much like an infection, and triggers an antibody response. In Hashimoto's, antibodies against the thyroid gland are produced, which interfere with its proper functioning. Like other forms of hypothyroidism, Hashimoto's usually requires long-term T4 therapy.

A diagnosis of Hashimoto's is confirmed by detecting specific thyroid antibodies in the blood. It is recommended that antibody testing be done on anyone experiencing fatigue and whose regular thyroid tests are normal. Fortunately, there are ways to help reduce thyroid antibodies and support thyroid health, and we'll explore some of those shortly.

REFLECTION POINT
In your journal, note whether any of the above situations apply to you. Double-check when your last thyroid blood work was done, and confirm that all the tests mentioned at the end of the chapter have been completed.

Complementary Therapies for Thyroid Dysfunction

Combined Prescription T4 and T3 Therapy

You learned about thyroid hormones in the opening section of this chapter, where you now know that two hormones are produced: T4 and T3. In most cases of low thyroid function or when the thyroid is removed, only T4 is prescribed. However, 15% of people may still experience persistent symptoms of low thyroid function, such as fatigue, feeling cold, and low mood [10].

Although not technically a complementary therapy, more people are now being treated with a combination of T4 and T3. In some individuals, T4 may not be sufficient to raise thyroid hormone levels adequately, and adding T3 can help achieve this goal [11]. T3 is a prescription medication; therefore, consult your doctor to determine if this approach is suitable for you.

Natural Therapies to Raise T4 and T3

Ashwagandha

This is one of my favorite herbs! Ashwagandha, also known as Indian Ginseng, is an Ayurvedic herb renowned for its multifaceted effects on the body and mind. It acts as an antioxidant, anti-inflammatory, antidepressant, and anti-anxiety agent, and even exhibits anticancer properties. Ashwagandha has been found to enhance sleep, boost energy, and support healthy thyroid function.

Ashwagandha can increase levels of T4 and T3 [12]. One reason Ashwagandha may have such an impact on the thyroid is due to its effect on another key hormone: cortisol. Numerous studies have found that Ashwagandha reduces cortisol levels [13]. Since high cortisol can impair thyroid function, stress reduction strategies like Ashwagandha may offer real benefits.

CLINICAL PEARL

To increase thyroid hormone levels, Ashwagandha can be safely taken for several months at doses of 500–600 mg. Note that if you have a thyroid storm or Graves' disease, you should avoid Ashwagandha.

Yoga

A consistent yoga practice has been shown to reduce cortisol levels, which in turn may help improve thyroid function. Remarkably, most people (and even many doctors) assume thyroid function can only improve with medication or supplements. However, mind-body practices like yoga, which incorporate slow breathing and mindful movements, have been found to increase T3 and T4 levels, resulting in a reduction in the need for medication [14].

Natural Therapies to Lower Antibody Levels

If you have had blood tests and it's confirmed that you have high thyroid antibody levels, lowering them is generally linked to an improvement in your condition. Interestingly, several natural therapies have been shown to decrease antibody levels and help restore healthy thyroid function.

Myo-inositol and Selenium

Not many people are aware of myo-inositol, but it can be found in foods such as certain vegetables and nuts. It plays an essential role in the production and signaling of several hormones, including thyroid hormones.

Selenium supports several antioxidant enzymes that help regulate inflammation throughout the body. When there is a selenium deficiency, these enzymes do not function properly, making the thyroid gland more vulnerable to immune dysfunction.

Multiple clinical trials have demonstrated that the combined supplementation of these two natural agents lowers antibody levels and restores thyroid hormone production [15], allowing the return of normal thyroid functioning [16].

CLINICAL PEARL

When antibodies are present, supplementing with 600 mg of myo-inositol and 80 mcg of selenium may help restore or improve thyroid function. Continue this protocol for 3–6 months.

Vitamin D

Low vitamin D levels are linked to an increased risk of autoimmune conditions [17]. Vitamin D is an essential nutrient for the body, playing a crucial role in immune function and thyroid health [18].

If antibodies are present, correction of vitamin D deficiency can bring these levels back within the normal range [19], improve thyroid function [20], and lessen fatigue.

> **CLINICAL PEARL**
>
> Aim for a serum vitamin D level of at least 80–150 nmol/L. You should check your vitamin D levels to determine the ideal daily intake. Vitamin D is measured through a simple blood test. Most recommendations for vitamin D intake range from 800 to 2,000 IU daily. However, if your vitamin D level is low, those doses may not be sufficient to increase your vitamin D levels.
>
> If your vitamin D level is below 70 nmol/L, I suggest taking 4,000 IU for three months, then retesting to confirm it has increased to the optimal level.

Nigella sativa Oil

Nigella sativa is the Latin name for what is commonly known as black seed oil, or black cumin oil. It's widely used as a culinary spice, especially in Middle Eastern cuisine.

In integrative medicine, black seed oil is valued for its antioxidant properties and notable benefits for thyroid health. Numerous clinical trials have found that supplementing with black seed oil reduces thyroid antibody levels and increases thyroid hormones [21].

> **CLINICAL PEARL**
>
> Try supplementing with *Nigella sativa* at a dose of 2–4 g per day for at least eight weeks to see the difference in your blood work.

Nutrition for Thyroid Health

Mediterranean Diet

By now, you are an expert on the Mediterranean diet and understand its key components. To review, this diet emphasizes healthy fats (such as fish, nuts, olive oil, and avocado), along with plenty of fruits, vegetables, and fiber-rich foods. It allows a modest intake of lean animal protein and limits or discourages the consumption of processed meats and processed foods.

This anti-inflammatory dietary approach helps lower thyroid antibody levels, leading to higher T4 and T3 levels, improved thyroid function, and increased energy [22].

Gluten-free Diet

Even if you don't have celiac disease, which is a condition where people cannot tolerate gluten, a gluten-free diet might benefit your thyroid health. Gluten is a protein found in wheat, barley, and rye that provides baked goods with their elasticity and texture. Some people experience digestive issues, such as bloating or constipation, when they eat gluten-containing foods.

One study found that a six-month gluten-free diet reduces antibody levels and improves vitamin D levels [23]. Another study found that a 12-month gluten-free diet improves thyroid hormone levels [24]. If you are struggling with fatigue and your thyroid is disrupted, try choosing gluten-free grains for at least six months. Good gluten-free options include rice, quinoa, buckwheat, and amaranth. Gluten can also hide in many packaged foods, so it's important to read ingredient labels carefully to ensure you're avoiding it completely.

CLINICAL PEARL

An acronym to remember grains that contain gluten, and that you may want to avoid, is BROWS-C: barley, rye, oats, wheat, spelt, and couscous.

Conclusion

Effective management of thyroid dysfunction in cancer survivors requires a collaborative approach that considers the patient's overall health. Combining complementary therapies, such as nutritional support, stress reduction, and herbal remedies, with standard treatments like T4 replacement can enhance thyroid care and support overall wellness. Managing cancer-related fatigue is a process, and acknowledging the importance of thyroid health is a crucial step toward renewed energy and an improved quality of life.

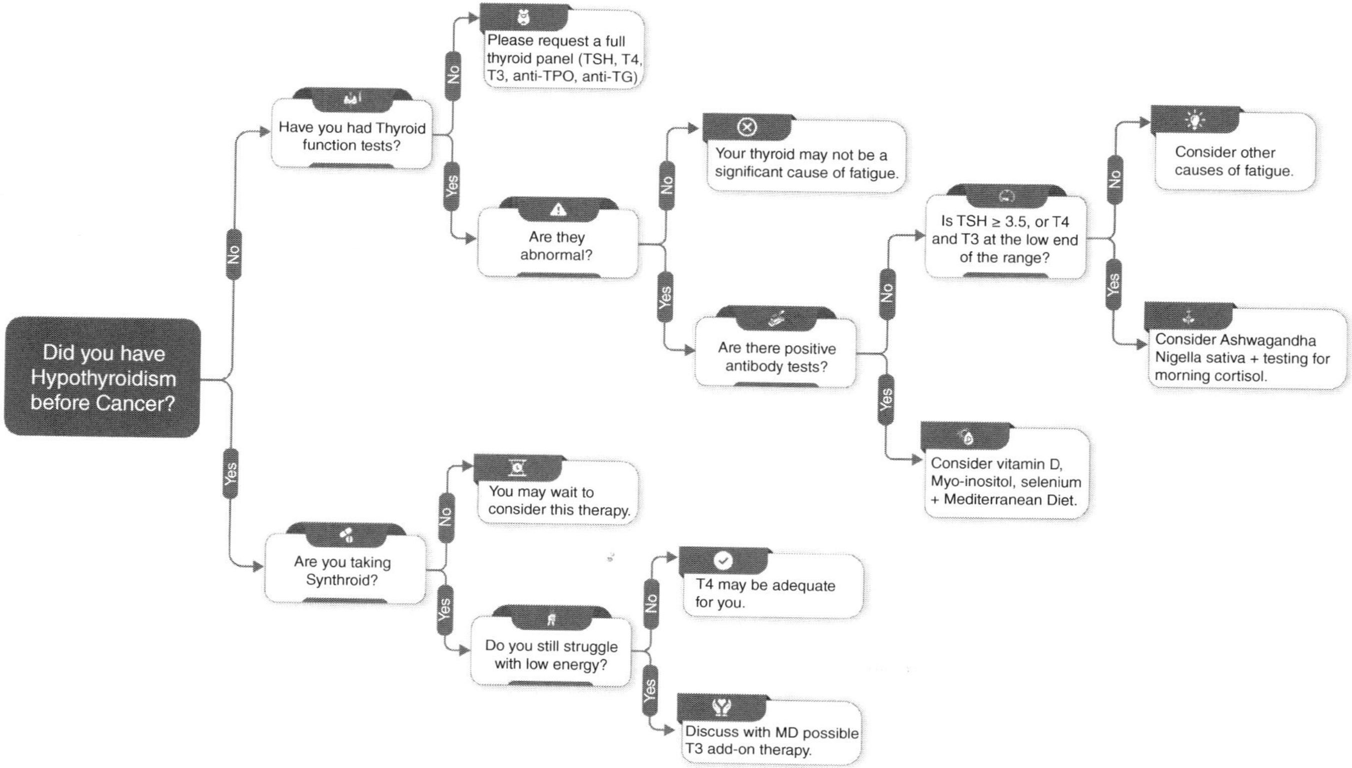
Did you have Hypothyroidism before Cancer?
No
Yes
Have you had Thyroid function tests?
No
Please request a full thyroid panel (TSH, T4, T3, anti-TPO, anti-TG)
Yes
Are they abnormal?
No
Your thyroid may not be a significant cause of fatigue.
Yes
Are there positive antibody tests?
No
Is TSH ≥ 3.5, or T4 and T3 at the low end of the range?
No
Consider other causes of fatigue.
Yes
Consider Ashwagandha Nigella sativa + testing for morning cortisol.
Yes
Consider vitamin D, Myo-inositol, selenium + Mediterranean Diet.
Are you taking Synthroid?
No
You may wait to consider this therapy.
Yes
Do you still struggle with low energy?
No
T4 may be adequate for you.
Yes
Discuss with MD possible T3 add-on therapy.

For Your Healthcare Practitioner

Routine thyroid assessments usually include thyroid-stimulating hormone (TSH), free T4, and free T3. However, it is worthwhile to consider adding thyroid antibody tests, specifically thyroglobulin antibody (TgAb) and thyroperoxidase antibody (TPOAb). These antibody tests are valuable and essential for determining if the thyroid might be contributing to fatigue, especially in symptomatic patients, even when standard thyroid tests fall within the normal range.

TgAb and TPOAb are frequently present in individuals with subclinical hypothyroidism, and their early detection can help prevent progression to overt thyroid dysfunction. Identifying these markers may also provide additional insights in cases where fatigue and other hypothyroid-like symptoms persist despite otherwise "normal" labs.

Unfortunately, although levothyroxine seems to regulate TSH and free T4 levels, this does not always lead to symptom relief or a better quality of life. Some studies suggest that, in such cases where TSH is normal and T4 alone is not effective, adding T3 therapy to levothyroxine may be a more successful approach [25].

For patients receiving immunotherapy, it may be possible to identify those at elevated risk for thyroid dysfunction. A study was conducted on 264 patients with various solid malignancies who received multiple ICI treatments. Baseline TgAb and TPOAb levels were tested, and while there were no differences between patients at the initiation of therapy, positive TPOAb and TgAb levels were both independent predictive factors and early biomarkers for the development of thyrotoxicosis [26]. This finding has been confirmed in other trials as well [27]. Although it is not yet the standard of care, consider a baseline screen for TgAb or TPOAb.

References

1 Maki Y, Horiuchi K, Okamoto T. Fatigue and quality of life among thyroid cancer survivors without persistent or recurrent disease. Endocr Connect, 2022; 11(2):e210506.

2 Ettleson MD, Bianco AC. Individualized therapy for hypothyroidism: is T4 therapy enough for everyone? J Clin Endocrinol Metab, 2020; 105(9):e3090–e3104.

3 Falstie-Jensen AM, Esen BO, Kjaersgaard A, et al. Incidence of hypothyroidism after treatment for breast cancer – a Danish matched cohort study. Breast Cancer Res, 2020; 22:106.

4 Marina D, Rasmussen AK, Buch-Larsen K, et al. Influence of the anti-oestrogens tamoxifen and letrozole on thyroid function in women with early and advanced breast cancer: a systematic review. Cancer Med, 2023; 12:967–982.
5 Brancatella A, Lupi I, Montanelli L, et al. Management of thyrotoxicosis induced by PD1 or PD-L1 blockade. J Endocr Soc, 2021; 5(9):bvab093.
6 Iwama S, Kobayashi T, Yasuda Y, et al. Increased risk of thyroid dysfunction by PD-1 and CTLA-4 blockade in patients without thyroid autoantibodies at baseline. J Clin Endocrinol Metab, 2022; 107:e1620.
7 Kudo M, Finn RS, Qin S, et al. Lenvatinib versus sorafenib in first-line treatment of patients with unresectable hepatocellular carcinoma: a randomized phase 3 non-inferiority trial. Lancet, 2018; 391(10126):1163–1173.
8 Kobayashi T, Iwama S, Yamagami A, et al. Combined use of tyrosine kinase inhibitors with PD-L1 blockade increased the risk of thyroid dysfunction in PD-L1 blockade: a prospective study. Cancer Immunol Immunother, 2024; 73:146.
9 Rooney MK, Andring LM, Corrigan KL, et al. Hypothyroidism following radiotherapy for head and neck cancer: a systematic review of the literature and opportunities to improve the therapeutic ratio. Cancers, 2023; 15(17):4321.
10 Wiersinga WM. T4 and T3 combination therapy: an unsolved problem of increasing magnitude and complexity. Endocrinol Metal, 2021; 36(5):938–951.
11 Tariq A, Wert Y, Cheriyath P, et al. Effects of long-term combination LT4 and LT3 therapy for improving hypothyroidism and overall quality of life. Sound Med J, 2018; 111(6):363–369.
12 Sharma AK, Basu I, Singh S. Efficacy and safety of Ashwagandha root extract in subclinical hypothyroid patients: a double-blind, randomized placebo-controlled trial. J Altern Complement Med, 2018; 24:243–248.
13 Wicinski M, Fajkiel-Madajczyk A, Kurant Z, et al. Can Ashwaghanda benefit the endocrine system? A review. Int J Mol Sci, 2023; 24(22):16513.
14 Bhandari RB, Mahto PK. Effect of yoga therapy on hypothyroidism: a systematic review. Ann Neurosci, 2024; 32(3):207–218.
15 Nordio M, Pajalich R. Combined treatment with Myo-inositol and selenium ensures euthyroidism in subclinical hypothyroidism patients with autoimmune thyroiditis. J Thyroid Res, 2013; 2013:424163.
16 Nordio M, Basciani S. Myo-inositol plus selenium supplementation restores euthyroid state in Hashimoto's patients with subclinical hypothyroidism. Eur Rev Med Pharmacol Sci, 2017; 21:51–59.
17 Heaney RP. Vitamin D in health and disease. Clin J Am Soc Nephrol, 2008; 3:1535–1541.
18 Soda M, Priante C, Pesce C, et al. The impact of vitamin D on immune function and its role in Hashimoto's thyroiditis: a narrative review. Life (Basel), 2024; 14(6):771.

19 Sulejmanovic M, Begic A, Mujaric-Bousbia F, et al. The relationship between thyroid antibodies and vitamin D levels in primary hypothyroidism. Med Arch, 2020; 74(5):359–362.

20 Muscogiuri G, Mari D, Prolo S, et al. 25-Hydroxyvitamin D deficiency and its relationship to autoimmune thyroid disease in the elderly. Int J Environ Res Public Health, 2016; 13:850.

21 Ghaffari-Saravi F, Jokar A. Herbal remedies for hypothyroidism: a systematic review and meta-analysis. Caspian J Intern Med, 2024; 16(1):1–8.

22 Ruggeri RM, Barbalace MC, Croce L, et al. Autoimmune thyroid disorders: the Mediterranean diet as a protective choice. Nutrients, 2023; 15(18):3953.

23 Krysiak R, Szkróbka W, Okopień B. The effect of gluten-free diet on thyroid autoimmunity in drug-naïve women with Hashimoto's thyroiditis: a pilot study. Exp Clin Endocrinol Diabetes, 2019; 127:417–422.

24 Pobłocki J, Pańka T, Szczuko M, et al. Whether a gluten-free diet should be recommended in chronic autoimmune thyroiditis or not?—a 12-month follow-up. J Clin Med, 2021; 10:3240.

25 Bunevicius R, Prange AJ. Mental improvement after replacement therapy with thyroxine plus triiodothyronine: relationship to cause of hypothyroidism. Int J Neuropsychopharmacol, 2000; 3(2):167–174.

26 Liu J, Chen M, Li S, et al. Biomarkers in the early stage of PD-1 inhibitor treatment have shown superior predictive capabilities for immune-related thyroid dysfunction. Front Immunol, 2024; 15:1458488.

27 Okada N, Iwama S, Okuji T, et al. Anti-thyroid antibodies and thyroid echo pattern at baseline as risk factors for thyroid dysfunction induced by anti-programmed cell death-1 antibodies: a prospective study. Br J Cancer, 2022; 122:771–777.

6

Estrogen: Finding Your Mojo After Menopause

When women take care of their health, they become their best friend

—Maya Angelou

It's not me, it's my hormones

—Women Everywhere

This chapter is for you if:

- You have a history of breast cancer, and you have been prescribed anti-estrogen hormone-blocking medications such as Tamoxifen or Letrozole/Anastrozole.
- You developed sudden menopausal symptoms following chemotherapy.
- You had your ovaries removed due to a gynecological cancer.
- You are in menopause and are experiencing fatigue.

From the first stirrings as a young woman, estrogen is one of the main hormones that orchestrates countless vital functions within our bodies. But with time, there is a gradual shift, estrogen levels naturally decline, and we enter the transition into menopause, bringing with it a host of physical and emotional changes.

Yet for many of those who have faced cancer, this gradual decline is accelerated, leaving women feeling plunged into menopause in an instant. Treatments such as chemotherapy, pelvic radiation, surgical removal of the ovaries, or hormone-blocking therapies can cause estrogen levels to drop earlier than expected. This can feel like being thrown into a whirlwind of hormonal changes all at once. Suddenly, you may find yourself dealing with mood swings, hot flashes, changes in weight or appetite, sleep disturbances, and profound fatigue. These don't feel like just changes, but more like an earthquake.

Beyond Cancer Fatigue: A Path to Reclaiming Energy, First Edition. Jessa Landmann, ND.

This isn't just in our minds or something we're making up! Estrogen has vital roles in our body, affecting our brain, bones, heart, and skin, creating a connected web of symptoms that can leave you feeling completely drained.

Understanding how estrogen influences these processes is empowering. It shows us that fatigue isn't just one thing; it's often a mix of factors. With this knowledge, the goal is to help you feel more informed, empowered, and to understand how everything works together. Let's take a closer look at how these processes operate and explore practical strategies you can use to feel more energized, one step at a time.

REFLECTION POINT
Get your journal ready, and start taking notes during this next section. Reflect on and record symptoms and side effects that you recognize as hindering your ability to feel your best.

Estrogen's Influence on The Regulation of Energy, Appetite and Weight

It's remarkable how powerfully estrogen supports us—helping to stabilize weight, balance appetite, and sustain vibrant energy from within. First, estrogen influences how the body processes and utilizes fat. It helps regulate fat cell activity—discouraging excess storage while promoting the breakdown of fat to create energy [1]. As estrogen levels decline, fat accumulates, often leading to elevated cholesterol levels [2].

Estrogen also influences how our body manages the sugars we eat. When our estrogen levels drop, this can lead to higher blood sugar levels, which can result in diabetes [3]. High cholesterol and high blood sugar can lead to weight gain, a slower metabolism, and contribute to the development of metabolic syndrome [4].

Excess fat can also accumulate in the muscles, leading to reduced muscle mass and increased muscular fatigue [5]. Our muscles play a significant role in determining how much energy and strength we have. When our muscles feel tired, we may want to exercise less, which can further contribute to muscle loss and increased fatigue.

Estrogen even plays a role in appetite regulation. It communicates with the brain's appetite centers to help you feel full after eating. After we eat, estrogen tells the brain to reduce food intake [6]. As estrogen levels decline, the brain receives fewer signals to stop eating [7]. The result is a reduced sense of fullness, a heightened appetite, and a greater tendency to store fat [8]. This is why gaining weight during menopause is so common, and weight gain is a well-recognized cause of fatigue.

As you can see, many systems are affected by estrogen, and they all work together. The good news is that understanding this big picture is one of the first and most essential steps toward reclaiming your energy.

Estrogen and Sleep

It is very common for cancer survivors to have sleep problems, especially women in menopause. Where maybe 2 out of 10 people in general experience sleep issues, it can be as high as 6 out of 10 for breast cancer survivors [9]. This isn't surprising when you think about all the ways menopause can affect you, like bothersome hot flashes, joint and muscle pain, and the need to urinate more frequently. Getting a good night's sleep is crucial for our overall health. Poor sleep is linked to poor memory and focus [10], lower survival rates, and an increased risk of cancer progression and recurrence [11].

One reason low estrogen can disrupt sleep is that it may suppress the regular release of melatonin, the hormone that regulates our sleep–wake cycle. This causes difficulty falling asleep, staying asleep, and early morning awakenings [12]. Melatonin levels typically decrease with age, and this decline may contribute to the menopause transition. Melatonin plays a role in bone health, which is also important for women [13].

It is also crucial to rule out sleep apnea. There is strong evidence that postmenopausal women face a higher risk of developing sleep apnea compared to premenopausal women [14]. People with sleep apnea often experience excessive daytime sleepiness, persistent insomnia, headaches, high blood pressure, impaired concentration, declining memory, and depression. Sound familiar? These symptoms are almost identical to those commonly seen in menopause. It's easy to see how sleep apnea can be overlooked or misdiagnosed in women going through menopause.

Sleep apnea is gaining attention because of its strong link to the development of cardiovascular disease, metabolic disorders like diabetes, and a decline in brain function [15]. Menopause and low estrogen already increase women's risk of these conditions, and if a woman has sleep apnea, this risk rises even more. That's why you may need to advocate for yourself to be screened for sleep apnea, especially if your doctor doesn't bring it up.

The good news is that there are many ways to improve sleep, and you deserve restful, rejuvenating sleep. Because sleep is so essential, Chapter 14 is devoted to it.

Estrogen and Changes in Cognition and Mood

It's truly remarkable how many systems in the body are affected by estrogen. Estrogen readily crosses the blood–brain barrier to support learning and memory. The area of the brain involved in these processes, known as the hippocampus, is rich in estrogen receptors. This explains why lowered estrogen from cancer treatments can lead to a feeling of brain fog, difficulty concentrating, poor memory, and poor word recall [16]. When the brain no longer receives its usual stimulation from estrogen, these symptoms can appear rapidly and noticeably.

Another factor to consider is exposure to chemotherapy. In breast cancer survivors who have undergone chemotherapy, up to 75% of women report a decreased ability to concentrate, remember, and think [17]. When given neurological testing, women who have been exposed to chemotherapy score poorly on language ability, verbal ability, working memory, and processing speed [18]. These challenges can significantly affect quality of life and are a major contributor to fatigue.

Beyond brain fog, changes in estrogen levels also affect our mood and emotional well-being. As estrogen levels decline, depression is one of the most common experiences for women, with about 35% of women feeling down [19]. Worry and anxiety are also widespread [20]. These emotions are typically associated with poorer sleep quality and increased fatigue. But as we'll explore in the chapters on depression and anxiety (Chapters 11 and 12), there are many tools available to help you feel more like yourself again.

Joint Pains

It is estimated that about 80% of women going through menopause will experience musculoskeletal pain [21]. They may report headaches, neck pain, back pain, hip discomfort, or knee pain—it can appear almost anywhere in the body. Joint pain interferes with the ability to get a good night's sleep, and pain tends to worsen when a woman is also depressed [22].

Joint and muscle pain affects nearly 50% of women being treated with an aromatase inhibitor, a drug used for estrogen-dominant breast cancer, and about 10% of women will cease their treatment because they cannot tolerate the pain [23].

Discontinuing cancer treatment increases the risk of recurrence and can reduce overall survival, which is why having effective strategies for managing pain is critical.

Hot Flashes

Astonishingly, up to 95% of women with low estrogen will experience hot flashes [24]. Estrogen helps maintain body temperature. Hot flashes occur because the drop in estrogen affects the hypothalamus, the part of the brain responsible for regulating body temperature and temperature regulation. The slightest change in temperature, often at night while women are sleeping, can trigger an overly sensitive response in the brain, resulting in sweating, which is often followed by feelings of cold and chills.

Hot flashes can be especially disruptive at night, disturbing sleep, and causing daytime drowsiness. Even when they occur during the day, hot flashes can significantly impact a woman's quality of life, leading to fatigue and low energy levels. If hot flashes are contributing to your fatigue, please know that you are not alone. Numerous complementary therapies can help alleviate these symptoms and support improved sleep and energy.

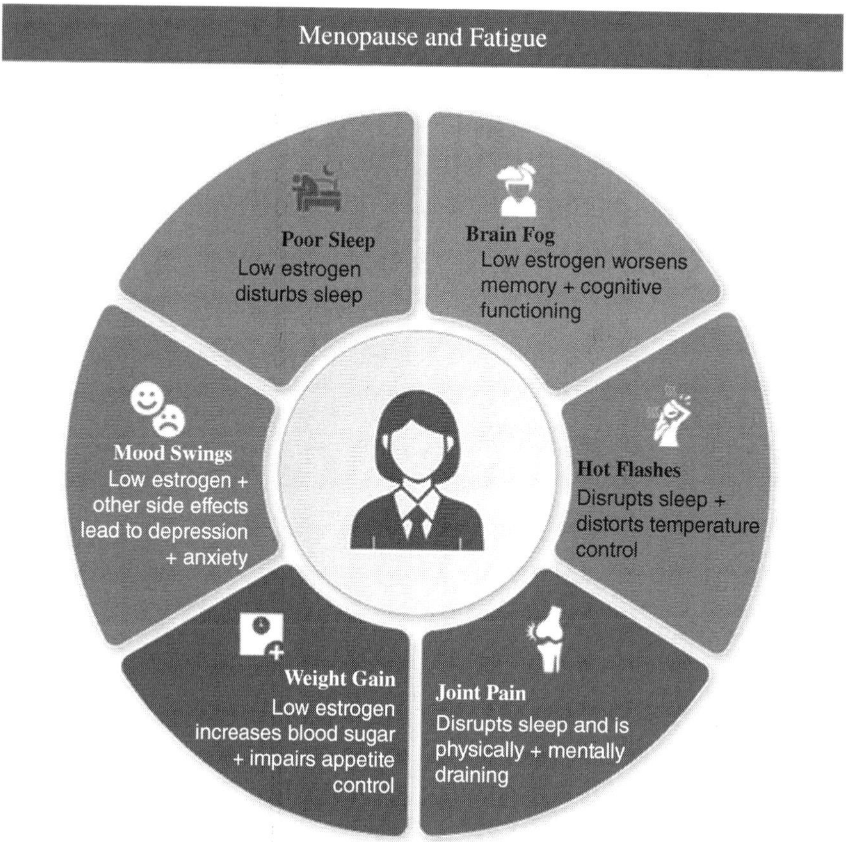

REFLECTION POINT

After all you have learned, jot down in your journal the aspects of menopause that seem to affect your energy the most. Do hot flashes and joint pain often awaken you? Do you notice cloudy thinking and find it upsetting? Has weight gain crept up on you, impacting your emotional health and leaving you tired? Are you constantly hungry, never feeling satisfied? As you list these, pay special attention to the suggestions in the next section and write down ideas for therapies you can try as soon as you finish reading.

Complementary Therapies to Combat the Effects of Low Estrogen and Fatigue

For women without a history of hormone-sensitive cancers, such as breast, endometrial, or ovarian cancer, oral hormone replacement therapy (HRT) is considered the gold standard for managing menopausal symptoms. HRT has been shown to improve sleep, reduce hot flashes, increase muscle mass, and improve body composition [25].

However, oral HRT is considered contraindicated in women with a history of hormone-driven cancers, as theoretically, extra estrogen could increase the risk of a recurrence [26]. This can understandably cause frustration, both among female cancer survivors and among family doctors, as most people do not know how else to manage menopausal symptoms.

So, how can you manage menopausal symptoms, boost energy, and feel more like yourself without HRT? That's precisely what the rest of this chapter aims to assist you with. Understanding the benefits of alternative therapies is essential. You might need to try a few different approaches to discover what works best for you. However, this guide will give you a starting point and improve your chances of success.

Strategies to Help Prevent Weight Gain

This book dedicates a whole chapter to weight loss, reviewing research on how to lose weight most effectively and which approaches are most successful. Interestingly, multiple eating patterns can support weight loss. It all comes down to what works for your preferences and what you can stick with. Please refer to Chapter 9 on weight loss for thorough guidance.

However, as a teaser, here are a few things commonly recommended to support energy and weight loss.

High Protein Intake

If there were one nutritional recommendation for all women, it would be to ensure they get enough protein. Beyond its role in weight loss, higher protein intake is one of the fastest ways to boost energy levels. There's an entire chapter 17 in this book devoted to meal planning and practical strategies to help you get enough protein each day, so be sure to check it out!

Women are notoriously protein deficient, and this has a significant impact on their muscle mass, energy levels, and sleep [27]. More muscle mass also boosts metabolism, which supports weight loss. A high-protein diet promotes feelings of fullness and reduces the drive to eat more. As you've learned, women with low estrogen may not get the same hunger/fullness cues, so a high-protein diet can help regulate appetite.

> **CLINICAL PEARL**
>
> To calculate how much protein you should be getting, take your ideal weight in kilograms, and multiply it by 1.2–1.5. This number represents the recommended amount of protein in grams you should aim for each day.

Exercise After a Meal

As discussed earlier, low estrogen levels can impair the body's ability to efficiently use dietary fats and sugars, often leading to elevated blood sugar and weight gain. However, we can hack this hormonal shift by engaging in light to moderate activity within 30 minutes of eating.

Walking after a meal can lower blood sugar levels and improve blood sugar control, ultimately reducing the risk of developing diabetes [28]. When we walk, our muscles are working, and this muscle activity takes up sugar from the bloodstream. This provides muscles with the energy they need and prevents the loss of muscle and muscular fatigue that we previously mentioned.

If you cannot get outside for a walk, you can walk around the area you are eating, down hallways, or up and down stairs. Aim for at least 10 minutes of movement after each meal. This small change can make a big difference in weight and energy management.

Complementary Therapies for Hot Flashes

There are many natural therapies available to help manage hot flashes. What works for one person might not work for another. You may have to try a few different strategies before finding what works best for you, but rest assured, relief is achievable. Let's look at some well-studied options.

Acupuncture

If you've never tried acupuncture before, now might be a great time to consider it. Of all the natural therapies that can help with hot flashes, acupuncture stands out as the one most consistently supported by research. It can reduce hot flashes in women on hormone therapy for breast cancer [29], as well as women who have gone through menopause for other reasons [30]. A noteworthy point is that acupuncture may be as effective as HRT for hot flashes [31].

Typical treatment regimens are given once or twice weekly for four to six weeks. Interestingly, even after acupuncture treatments are finished, their effects can last for several months.

CLINICAL PEARL

My acupuncture protocol for hot flashes includes the following points: LV2, KI3, SP6, ST36, CV4, HT7, LI4, LI11, Shenmen, and GV20. Feel free to show this to your acupuncturist; they'll know exactly what it means!

Herbal Therapies and Supplements

Soy

Soy products have long been surrounded by controversy, especially regarding estrogen-sensitive cancers. However, increasing research suggests that soy is, in fact, safe for women with estrogen-driven cancers and does not raise the risk of developing or worsening cancer [32]. Soy is just one type of food or herbal product called a phytoestrogen. A phytoestrogen is a compound found in plant-based foods, such as soy, flax, and grains, that resembles estrogen and can help alleviate some symptoms associated with low estrogen levels.

Regarding hot flashes, soy may be effective for some women [33, 34]. It is generally considered safe for long-term use, with no unwanted effects on the breast, uterus, or liver [35]. Additionally, despite the historical controversy that phytoestrogens increase estrogen in the blood, it has not been found to do so [36].

CLINICAL PEARL

When looking for a supplement, you will be searching for a product labelled "soy isoflavones." The doses studied vary widely, ranging from 30 to 75 mg twice daily. You may have to experiment with the dose that works for you, so start at 30 mg per day and work your way up to 75 mg twice per day.

Black Cohosh

Black cohosh is another plant-based therapy that, like soy, is classified as a phytoestrogen. A recent large-scale meta-analysis found that black cohosh, overall, is effective for hot flashes [37]. However, to be completely transparent, this hasn't always been the case [38].

In terms of safety, black cohosh does not elevate estrogen levels, nor does it cause any liver damage [39]. Women need to know which complementary options are safe to try, especially when managing symptoms like hot flashes, disrupted sleep, and fatigue. If you've tried other remedies without success, this may be worth exploring.

CLINICAL PEARL

Doses in clinical trials vary, but the recommended starting dose is 40 mg to 150 mg of black cohosh per day.

Valerian

This herb is often included in formulas or teas that promote relaxation, reduce stress, and improve sleep. It is not well known for hot flashes, as only a few clinical trials have been conducted [40]. However, this is one of my favorites, especially as a supplement. I often recommend it more than soy or black cohosh supplements, as I have had the most success with it.

CLINICAL PEARL

Dosing varies in research studies, but I recommend 300 mg in capsule form, taken three or four times daily (breakfast, lunch, dinner, and before bed).

Complementary Therapies for Sleep

Helping someone achieve restful sleep is fascinating because it often reveals a beautiful truth common in medicine: solving one issue usually improves many others. Take hot flashes, for example. If a woman is repeatedly jolted awake by the heat of sweating, helping alleviate those bothersome hot flashes should, by default, improve her sleep. The same goes for joint or muscle pain. Alleviating pain not only improves comfort but also naturally leads to better, deeper sleep.

This is the beauty of integrative medicine. It's not about chasing symptoms but about identifying the root causes of the struggle. Once that core issue is addressed, a remarkable domino effect often follows.

To avoid repetition, a complete discussion of sleep strategies, including sleep hygiene, herbal options, acupuncture, and nutritional approaches, can be found in Chapter 14.

Complementary Therapies for Brain Fog

Acupuncture

Several nerves on the scalp and head can be stimulated through acupuncture. Acupuncture has been shown to increase a protein called brain-derived neurotrophic factor (BDNF), which plays a crucial role in the survival and growth of nerve cells in the brain. Increasing BDNF helps to improve memory, learning, and may help treat a variety of cognitive and mental disorders, such as Alzheimer's and depression [41].

Numerous studies have demonstrated that acupuncture produces significant improvements in cognitive functioning [42]. Acupuncture may be as effective as cognitive behavioral therapy for cognition [43]. Fascinatingly, acupuncture may stop the breakdown of brain tissue, and improvements in brain structure have been found on MRI after acupuncture [44].

CLINICAL PEARL

My acupuncture protocol for cognitive impairment is as follows: Sishencong, GV20, GV24, GB20, HT7, PC6, KD3, and ST36. Show this to your acupuncturist, and leave the needles in for 30 minutes, twice per week, for six to eight weeks.

Lion's Mane

Lion's mane is a medicinal mushroom that has been studied in people with early-onset Alzheimer's disease and mild cognitive impairment, and has been found to improve symptoms [45]. My experience with Lion's Mane in clinical practice has been positive in helping women feel clearer and less foggy. My patients report better word recall and better memory.

CLINICAL PEARL
Try 1,000 mg of Lion's Mane extract for at least three months.

Cardiovascular Exercise

Aerobic exercise consistently improves cognitive functioning, particularly in areas such as processing speed, memory, and attention. Cardiovascular activity increases the flow of oxygen-rich blood to the brain, boosting the performance of brain cells. In breast cancer survivors who have undergone chemotherapy and experience brain fog, cardiovascular exercise has proven to alleviate their symptoms [46]. Exercise also improves sleep, increases energy levels, and enhances overall quality of life.

CLINICAL PEARL
Here's a simple-to-follow protocol you can do anywhere. It involves a 30-second high-intensity exercise with maximum effort, then a 1-minute rest. The exercises include jumping jacks, high knees, jump squats, burpees, and speed skaters. Do each for 30 seconds, rest for one minute, and repeat for two or three rounds. Aim to do this five days a week.

Fruit and Vegetables

One of the leading causes of brain fog after chemotherapy is inflammation in the brain. Therefore, anti-inflammatories can help relieve these symptoms. A simple yet effective method is through diet. Fruits and vegetables are rich in antioxidants and decrease inflammation. Research suggests that increasing fruit and vegetable intake (two servings of fruit and four servings of vegetables daily) improves symptoms of cognitive dysfunction [47].

Omega-3 Fatty Acids

Omega-3 fats, found in oily fish and available in supplement form, cross into the brain and have powerful anti-inflammatory properties [48]. Omega-3 fats, particularly when combined with a low-sugar diet, are beneficial for memory [49].

While some brain-boosting interventions, such as Lion's Mane or cardio, may offer quicker results, omega-3s typically take time to show their full benefits. If you decide to try them, stick with them for at least four months.

CLINICAL PEARL

When taking an omega-3 supplement, aim for at least 2 g of combined EPA and DHA. Check the label for the exact dosage of these fatty acids, and make sure to take the correct amount of both.

Complementary Therapies for Joint Pain

Chapter 15 is dedicated to managing various types of pain through complementary therapies. To avoid excessive repetition, please refer to that chapter for a thorough review of pain management techniques available. For joint pain, you'll discover that acupuncture and physical activity are highly effective.

Special Note on Vaginal Estrogen

Although oral HRT may not be recommended for breast cancer survivors to manage menopausal symptoms, vaginal estrogen is an approved, safe, and effective treatment for genitourinary conditions. Many women going through menopause experience vaginal dryness, pain during intercourse, frequent urinary tract infections, and the need to urinate often.

While these vaginal symptoms may not significantly contribute to fatigue, they impact quality of life. Vaginal estrogen is effective for increasing the vagina's natural lubrication and may boost sexual desire. It also improves vaginal elasticity, making sex more enjoyable and reducing pain. Additionally, vaginal estrogen decreases the frequency of urinary tract infections by approximately 50% [50].

Breast cancer survivors need not worry that exposure to estrogen will lead to cancer recurrence. The American Society of Clinical Oncology (ASCO) recently shared its findings that women with a history of breast cancer who used vaginal estrogen had better survival rates than those who did not. This is a groundbreaking discovery that could change how menopause is managed for cancer survivors and help many women regain comfort, confidence, and quality of life.

Success Story

Constance, a 47-year-old mother of two, came to see me as a patient three months after completing her chemotherapy. Her primary concern was fatigue. She had early-stage breast cancer but had a positive lymph node after her lumpectomy and underwent six cycles of chemotherapy. She also started Tamoxifen since her cancer tested estrogen-positive.

She was feeling very hopeful about her prognosis, but struggled with the effects of sudden menopause. She told me her hot flashes were not too severe and that she woke once at night from a hot flash. Her main sleep issue was her hip pain, which started after chemo and Tamoxifen treatment. She could not find a comfortable position to sleep and was frequently awakened by her pain.

Her other main complaints were constipation and muscle weakness. She used to be very active and used to lift weights at the gym four times a week. However, she now feels too tired to work out. Her constipation has persisted since chemotherapy, and every few days, she needs to take a laxative for relief.

We ran some blood tests and found that her thyroid function was low (T4 and T3 were at the lower end of the reference range), and her inflammation markers were high (CRP was 15.5), which was expected since she had recently finished her cancer treatment.

I recommended acupuncture to help with the hip pain, constipation, and hot flashes. We started herbal therapy with Ashwagandha for thyroid support (see Chapter 5), and I advised her to adopt the Mediterranean diet to reduce inflammation. I also emphasized the importance of resuming strength training three days a week, even for just 10 minutes each day, to prevent muscle loss.

After two acupuncture treatments, her bowel movements became regular, her hip pain lessened, her hot flashes vanished, and she was sleeping through the night. She followed the nutrition and exercise advice. However, she still felt muscle weakness, like her legs might give way.

We conducted additional tests for insulin resistance (fasting glucose and fasting insulin, see Chapter 8 *on diabetes), and we found that her HOMA-IR score was elevated. Upon closer review of her dietary habits, it was observed that she consumed a high amount of sweets as a stress-relief mechanism and dined out at fast food restaurants at least three times per week.*

We changed her diet to a high-protein, very low-carbohydrate eating pattern. I also explained that processed foods are linked to low energy levels and advised avoiding fast food whenever possible. After one month of maintaining this diet and exercising, while limiting carbs to only fruits and vegetables, she noticed a significant boost in her muscle strength and energy levels.

We tested her thyroid hormone levels and inflammation again three months later. Both her T4 and T3 improved, and her inflammation decreased (CRP was 2.1). She initially rated her energy at 4/10, and now she rates it at 9/10.

References

1 D'Eon TM, Souza SC, Aronovitz M, et al. Estrogen regulation of adiposity and fuel partitioning. Evidence of genomic and non-genomic regulation of lipogenic and oxidative pathways. J Biol Chem, 2005; 280:35983–35991.
2 Currie H, Williams C. Menopause, cholesterol and cardiovascular disease. US Cardiology, 2008; 5(1):12–14.
3 Louet J-F, LeMay C, Mauvais-Jarvis F. Anti-diabetic actions of estrogen: insight from human and genetic mouse models. Curr Atheroscler Rep, 2004; 6:180–185.
4 Musatov S, Chen W, Pfaff DW, et al. Silencing of estrogen receptor α in the ventromedial nucleus of hypothalamus leads to metabolic syndrome. Proc Natl Acad Sci USA, 2007; 104:2501–2506.
5 Zhang C, Feng X, Zhang X, et al. Research progress on the correlation between estrogen and estrogen receptor on postmenopausal sarcopenia. Front Endocrinol, 2024; 15:1494972.
6 Palmer K, Gray JM. Central vs peripheral effects of estrogen on food intake and lipoprotein lipase activity in ovariectomized rats. Physiol Behav, 1986; 37:187–189.
7 Pfaff D, Keiner M. Atlas of estradiol-concentrating cells in the central nervous system of the female rat. J Comp Neurol, 1973; 151:121–158.
8 Gao Q, Horvath T. Cross-talk between estrogen and leptin signalling in the hypothalamus. Am J Physiol Endocrinol Metab, 2008; 294(5):817–826.
9 Ford ES, Cunningham TJ, Giles WH, et al. Trends in insomnia and excessive daytime sleepiness among US adults from 2002 to 2012. Sleep Med, 2015; 16(3):372–378.
10 Van Dyk K, Bower JE, Crespi CM, et al. Cognitive function following breast cancer treatment and associations with concurrent symptoms. Breast Cancer, 2018; 4(1):25.
11 Sephton S, Spiegel D. Circadian disruption in cancer: a neuroendocrine-immune pathway from stress to disease? Brain Behav Immun, 2003; 17(5):321–328.
12 Toffol E, Kalleinen N, Haukka J, et al. Melatonin in perimenopausal and postmenopausal women: associations with mood, sleep, climacteric symptoms, and quality of life. Menopause, 2014; 21(5):493–500.
13 Kotlarczyk MP, Lassila HC, O'Neil CK, et al. Melatonin osteoporosis prevention study (MOPS): a randomized, double-blind, placebo-controlled study examining the effects of melatonin on bone health and quality of life in perimenopausal women. J Pineal Res, 2012; 52(4):414–426.
14 Perger E, Mattaliano P, Lombardi C. Menopause and sleep apnea. Maturitas, 2019; 124:35–38.
15 Fietze I, Laharnar N, Bargiotas P, et al. Management of obstructive sleep apnea in Europe–a 10-year follow-up. Sleep Med, 2022; 97:64–72.

16 Maki PM, Jeff NG. Menopause and brain fog: how to counsel and treat midlife women. Menopause, 2024; 31(7):647–649.

17 Janelsins MC, Heckler CE, Peppone LJ, et al. Cognitive complaints in survivors of breast cancer after chemotherapy compared with age-matched controls: an analysis from a nationwide, multicenter prospective longitudinal study. J Clin Oncol, 2017; 35(5):506–514.

18 Bernstein LJ, McCreath GA, Komeylian Z, et al. Cognitive impairment in breast cancer survivors treated with chemotherapy depends on control group type and cognitive domains assessed: a multilevel meta-analysis. Neurosci Biobehav Rev, 2017; 83:417–428.

19 Jia Y, Zhou Z, Xiang F, et al. Global prevalence of depression in menopausal women: a systematic review and meta-analysis. J Affect Disord, 2024; 358:474–482.

20 Zhao R, Liu H, Gao J. Side effects of endocrine therapy are associated with depression and anxiety in breast cancer patients accepting endocrine therapy: a cross-sectional study in China. Front Psychol, 2022; 13:905459.

21 Lu C, Liu P, Zhou Y, et al. Musculoskeletal pain during the menopausal transition: a systematic review and meta-analysis. Neural Plast, 2020; 2020:8842110.

22 Frange C, Hachul H, Hirotsu C, et al. Insomnia with musculoskeletal pain in postmenopause: associations with symptoms, mood, and quality of life. J Menopausal Med, 2018; 24(1):17–28.

23 Kim S, Chen N, Reid, P. Current and future advances in practice: aromatase-inhibitor induced arthralgia. Rheumatol Adv Pract, 2024; 8(2):rkae024.

24 Cole KM, Clemons M, Alzahrani M, et al. Vasomotor symptoms in early breast cancer – a real world exploration of the patient experience. Support Care Cancer, 2022; 30:4437–4446.

25 Kleis-Olsen AS, Farlov JE, Petersen EA, et al. Metabolic flexibility in postmenopausal women: hormone replacement therapy is associated with higher mitochondrial content, respiratory capacity, and lower total fat mass. Acta Physiol, 2024; 240(6):e14117.

26 Holmberg L, Iversen O-E, Rudenstam CM, et al. Increased risk of recurrence after hormone replacement therapy in breast cancer survivors. J Natl Cancer Inst, 2008; 100(7):475–482.

27 Zhou J, Kim JE, Armstrong CL, et al. Higher protein diets improve indexes of sleep in energy-restricted overweight and obese adults: results from 2 randomized controlled trials. Am J Clin Nutr, 2016; 103(3):766–774.

28 Engeroff T, Groneberg DA, Wilke J. After dinner rest a while, after supper walk a mile? A systematic review with meta-analysis on the acute postprandial glycemic response to exercise before and after a meal ingestion in healthy subjects and patients with impaired glucose tolerance. Sports Med, 2023; 53(4):849–869.

29 Serra D, Fleishman SB, White C, et al. Acupuncture reduces severity of hot flashes in breast cancer: a randomized single-blind trial. Holist Nurs Pract, 2023; 37(6):330–336.

30 Soares JM, Branco-de-Luca AC, da Fonseca AM, et al. Acupuncture ameliorated vasomotor symptoms during menopausal transition: single-blind, placebo-controlled randomized trial to test treatment efficacy. Menopause, 2020; 28(1):80–85.

31 Palma F, Fontanesi F, Facchinetti F, et al. Acupuncture or phytoestrogens vs. estrogen plus progestin on menopausal symptoms: a randomized study. Gynecol Endocrinol, 2019; 35(11):995–998.

32 Guha N, Kwan ML, Quesenberry CP Jr, et al. Soy isoflavones and risk of cancer recurrence in a cohort of breast cancer survivors: the Life After Cancer Epidemiology study. Breast Cancer Res Treat, 2009; 118(2):395–405.

33 Palma F, Fontanesi F, Neri I, et al. Blood pressure and cardiovascular risk factors in women treated for climacteric symptoms with acupuncture, phytoestrogens or hormones. Menopause, 2020; 27(9):1060–1065.

34 Ye Y, Wang Z, Zhuo S, et al. Soy germ isoflavones improve menopausal symptoms but have no effect on blood lipids in postmenopausal Chinese women: a randomized placebo-controlled trial. Menopause, 2012; 19(7):791–798.

35 Colacurci N, De Franciscis P, Atlante M, et al. Endometrial, breast and liver safety of soy isoflavones plus *Lactobacillus sporogenes* in post menopausal women. Gynecol Endocrinol, 2013; 29(3):209–212.

36 Reed SD, Newton KM, LaCroix AZ, et al. Vaginal, endometrial, and reproductive hormone findings: randomized, placebo-controlled trial of black cohosh, multibotanical herbs and dietary soy for vasomotor symptoms: the Herbal Alternative for Menopause (HALT) study. Menopause, 2008; 15(1):51–58.

37 Hedaoo K, Badge AK, Tirade Y, et al. Exploring the efficacy and safety of black cohosh (*Cimicifuga racemosa*) in menopausal symptom management. J Midlife Health, 2024; 15(1):5–11.

38 Geller SE, Shulman LP, van Breeman RB, et al. Safety and efficacy of black cohosh and red clover for the management of vasomotor symptoms: a randomized controlled trial. Menopause, 2009; 16(6):1156–1166.

39 Nasr A, Naffed H. Influence of black cohosh (*Cimicifuga racemosa*) on postmenopausal women on total hepatic perfusion and liver functions. Fertil Steril, 2009; 92(5):1780–1782.

40 Jenabi E, Shobeiri F, Hazavehei S, et al. The effect of valerian on the severity and frequency of hot flashes: a triple-blind randomized clinical trial. Women Health, 2018; 58(3):297–304.

41 Yiyi L, Fang L, Dongdong Q, et al. The role of brain-derived neurotrophic factor in central nervous system. Front Aging Neurosci, 2022; 14:986443.

42 Li X, Lampson K, Ahles TA, et al. Feasibility and preliminary effects of acupuncture on cognitive dysfunction in divers cancer survivors: a pilot, randomized, placebo controlled trial. Curr Oncol, 2025; 32(1):27.

43 Liou KT, Garland SN, Li QS, et al. Effects of acupuncture virus cognitive behavioural therapy on brain-derived neurotrophic factor in cancer survivors with insomnia: an exploratory analysis. Acupunct Med, 2021; 39(6):637–645.

44 Zeng Y, Cheng ASK, Song T, et al. Effects of acupuncture on cancer-related cognitive impairment in Chinese gynecological cancer patients: a pilot court study. Integr Cancer Ther, 2018; 17(3):737–746.

45 Li IC, Chang HH, Lin CH, et al. Prevention of early Alzheimer's disease by Erinacine A-enriched *Hericium erinaceus* mycelia pilot double-line placebo-controlled study. Front Aging Neurosci, 2020; 12:155.

46 Hartman SJ, Nelson SH, Myers E, et al. Randomized controlled trial of increasing physical activity on objectively measured and self-reported cognitive functioning among breast cancer survivors: the memory & motion study. Cancer, 2018; 124(1):192–202.

47 Zuniga K, Moran N. Low serum carotenoids are associated with self-reported cognitive dysfunction and inflammatory markers in breast cancer survivors. Nutrients, 2018; 10(8):1111.

48 Dyall SC. Long-chain omega-3 fatty acids and the brain: a review of the independent and shared effects of EPA, DPA and DHA. Front Aging Neurosci, 2015; 7:52.

49 Orchard TS, Gaudier-Diaz MM, Weinhold KR, et al. Clearing the fog: a review of the effects of dietary omega-3 fatty acids and added sugars on chemotherapy-induced cognitive deficits. Breast Cancer Res Treat, 2017; 161(3):391–398.

50 Tan-Kim J, Shah NM, Do D, et al. Efficacy of vaginal estrogen for recurrent urinary tract infection prevention in hypoestrogenic women. Am J Obstet Gynecol, 2023; 229(2):143.

7

Testosterone: Vitality After Prostate Cancer

It takes more courage to reveal insecurities than to hide them, more strength to relate to people than to dominate them, more "manhood" to abide by thought-out principles rather than blind reflex. Toughness is in the soul and spirit, not in muscles and an immature mind

—Alex Karras, athlete

This chapter is for you if:

- You were diagnosed with prostate cancer and underwent a prostatectomy to remove the prostate surgically.
- You have undergone treatment for prostate cancer, which may include chemotherapy, radiation therapy, or androgen deprivation therapy.

Prostate cancer is the most commonly diagnosed cancer among men, touching countless lives. While navigating a diagnosis and the aftermath of treatments, a challenge often emerges in the form of a deep, pervasive fatigue, reported by a staggering 25–90% of men [1]. Fatigue in these men is a complex symptom, woven from a unique web of physical and emotional side effects linked directly to specific treatments like surgery, radiation, or androgen deprivation therapy (ADT).

But you don't have to live with this fatigue. This chapter serves as your guide to understanding the intricate factors that contribute to it, providing clear insights and practical, targeted strategies to help you reclaim your vitality. We'll explore how specific treatments can impact your energy and, most importantly, provide you with actionable steps to navigate your path to renewed strength. To help you visualize this journey, we've included a straightforward flowchart at the end of this chapter, designed to illuminate the road toward healing and lasting energy.

Fatigue stems from a variety of treatment-related causes. In cases where the cancer is confined to the prostate, a prostatectomy is the best option. While often

Beyond Cancer Fatigue: A Path to Reclaiming Energy, First Edition. Jessa Landmann, ND.

effective, the anesthesia, post-operative pain, and the emotional impact of surgery can contribute to fatigue. Longer-term side effects, such as urinary leakage or erectile dysfunction, may cause emotional distress and affect your overall quality of life, which can also lead to fatigue [2].

Radiation therapy is another common treatment for localized prostate cancer. The treatment protocol is intensive and may cause significant side effects affecting energy, including bladder pain, bowel issues such as diarrhea, and rectal pain.

Among all treatment options, men undergoing ADT often face the most significant challenges with energy. ADT suppresses testosterone production and can cause a range of side effects: hot flashes (which disrupt sleep), weight gain, loss of muscle mass, high blood sugar, feelings of depression, reduced sex drive, and insomnia [3]. Each of these symptoms causes, contributes to or worsens fatigue.

Navigating life after prostate cancer can be challenging. The following pages offer evidence-based strategies to help you manage side effects and regain your energy.

Side Effects of Prostatectomy

Complementary Therapies for Urinary Incontinence

Urinary incontinence refers to poor bladder control that can occur after surgery. Like many surgical procedures, prostatectomy carries risks, including possible nerve damage or weakened pelvic muscles, both of which may affect your ability to hold urine.

Urinary incontinence can lead to fatigue due to frequent nighttime awakenings. Men may wake up because of the urge to urinate or because they feel wet and cold if they experience leakage during sleep. The emotional distress caused by this side effect also contributes to mental fatigue and anxiety [4].

The good news is that 80–95% of men regain complete bladder control within one year of surgery. For some, this recovery can take up to two years [5]. If you are among those still struggling with urinary incontinence for longer, here are some therapies that can help.

Kegel Exercises

Kegel exercises, also known as pelvic floor exercises, involve contracting and relaxing the muscles that control the flow of urine. To find the right muscles, try stopping your urine stream a few times while urinating. Another way to locate these muscles is to imagine trying to stop passing gas. Practice contracting these muscles a few times, and if you feel tightening in your rectal area, you are engaging the correct muscles.

Incorporate Kegel exercises into your daily routine; it takes just five minutes. Contract your pelvic muscles, hold for three seconds, then release. Repeat this sequence 15 times, ensuring that you do not engage the muscles in your glutes. Evidence suggests that the earlier you start, the more likely it is to fully restore urinary function with just Kegels.

Acupuncture

When nerve damage is suspected, acupuncture should be considered as a primary treatment option. Research indicates that acupuncture stimulates the nervous system and can promote the healing and potential regrowth of damaged nerves [6]. Multiple studies suggest that acupuncture improves urinary incontinence after prostatectomy. When combined with Kegels, results may be achieved more quickly.

You might feel worried and wonder: where do the acupuncture needles go? The nerves that control the bladder originate from the lower back and sacral region. Needles are usually placed in these areas and connected to a low-frequency electrical current for therapeutic stimulation.

CLINICAL PEARL

Show this protocol to your acupuncturist:

The nerves that control bladder function exit the spinal cord at T12, L1, and L2 levels of the spine, as well as the foramina of S2, S3, and S4. Use Jiaji points T12-L2 and BL31-34 acupoints. Insert needles to a depth of 0.5 cun and apply electroacupuncture at 2 Hz for 30 minutes, twice weekly, for 10–12 sessions.

Success Story

Peter came to see me nine months after his prostate removal due to prostate cancer. He was still struggling with urinary incontinence, despite regularly doing Kegel exercises. He found that he woke up frequently at night to change his urinary pad, often awakening with a feeling of cold and wetness. He also found it difficult to fall back asleep once he was woken and reported getting about four to five hours of sleep, leaving him feeling very tired. He rated his energy at 3/10.

Peter also told me he was feeling depressed. He was an enthusiastic golfer in his retirement, spending about five days a week on the golf course with his friends. While golfing, he worried that his urinary pad might leak, which caused him significant distress. He usually needed to change his pad roughly four times a day.

He was used to walking the entire course, but since standing upright worsened his urinary leakage, he started driving the course instead, which meant missing out on conversations and laughter with his friends.

Peter also noticed that because he was walking significantly less, he had gained weight. We examined his dietary intake and found that he was consuming more sweets and candy than usual, and was eating later at night. He admitted to stress eating and recognized he needed to make some changes.

We talked about how acupuncture might help reduce urinary leakage, and he decided to try it. After just three sessions, he realized he wasn't waking during the night at all. Surprisingly, when he woke in the morning, his pad was completely dry. However, he didn't notice any changes during the day.

We also discussed how weight gain might increase pressure on the bladder, leading to more frequent urination. We allowed him to indulge his sweet tooth, but instead of sweets and candy, he replaced those treats with a high-protein fruit smoothie twice daily, as a high-protein diet supports weight loss and reduces appetite.

We continued the acupuncture for six more sessions, and after one month of careful avoidance of sweets, Peter lost 10 pounds. He noticed an improvement in his daytime urinary leakage, and he only had to change his pad once a day.

He felt more confident, was walking the course again, and after two months, he rated his energy at an 8/10.

Complementary Therapies for Erectile Dysfunction

Surgeons are increasingly successful at preserving nerve function during prostatectomy, and rates of complete erectile dysfunction have improved over the years. Some men can regain sexual function naturally with time. Medications like Viagra are commonly prescribed and can help [7]. If you're seeking additional support in this area, some complementary therapies may also be beneficial.

Kegel Exercises

Like urinary incontinence, strengthening your pelvic floor muscles can also help reduce erectile dysfunction [8]. There is also some evidence indicating that Kegels may enhance the quality of your orgasms. If that gives you a little extra motivation, all the better to keep at it!

Acupuncture

Although research is still emerging, acupuncture remains a promising complementary treatment for erectile dysfunction. The nerves that control bladder function also support sexual function, so acupuncture aimed at these areas may provide dual benefits. You can show your acupuncturist the bladder-focused protocol mentioned earlier in this chapter, as it might also be relevant here.

Side Effects of Radiation Therapy

Radiation therapy is a highly effective cancer treatment for targeting cancer cells, but it can also harm nearby tissue. In prostate cancer treatment, the most commonly affected adjacent tissues are the bladder and the bowel.

This collateral damage can irritate the bladder, leading to symptoms like pain during urination, bladder spasms, increased urinary frequency, and urgency. Up to 16% of men may have pain in the urethra, even many years later [9]. Damage to the bowel can cause pain, diarrhea, and cramping. These side effects can be disruptive to daily life, interfere with sleep, contribute to emotional distress, and lead to extreme fatigue. Let's examine some therapies that can help alleviate these symptoms.

Complementary Therapies for Radiation-induced Cystitis (Inflammation of the Bladder)

Hyperbaric Oxygen Therapy (HBOT)

Depending on your location, access to a hyperbaric oxygen chamber may not be readily available; however, if it is, this therapy is worth considering. HBOT involves resting in a chamber that delivers oxygen to deeper tissues to promote increased blood flow and healing. This significantly reduces the severity of symptoms, and these benefits can persist for up to five years following treatment [10].

Complementary Therapies for Diarrhea

Gastrointestinal complaints are common after pelvic radiation. Up to 33% of men report long-term symptoms like cramping, diarrhea, and rectal urgency (feeling like they can't "hold it") after radiation [11]. However, diarrhea can occur months to years later, leading to watery stools, abdominal pain, and bloating [12]. Chronic diarrhea can result in nutritional deficiencies, dehydration, and ultimately fatigue.

Some men turn to over-the-counter medications like Imodium, which can provide short-term relief. However, these treatments can have the opposite effect, causing constipation, leading men to feel trapped in a vicious cycle of diarrhea followed by constipation. Here's a more balanced approach.

Nutritional Interventions

While it makes logical sense that dietary changes could help manage these symptoms, research has not yet identified any clear guidelines. In my clinical experience, the Mediterranean diet remains the most supportive choice. It's healthy, anti-inflammatory, avoids processed foods, and can be effective for decreasing the severity of radiation-related diarrhea [13].

Probiotics

Probiotics are live "friendly" bacteria that support gut health. They help regulate digestion, and they can reduce inflammation. Radiation therapy disturbs the bacteria in our gut, which is a key reason why diarrhea occurs after pelvic radiation [14]. An extensive research review concluded that specific combinations of probiotic strains can be effective in reducing radiation-induced diarrhea [15].

CLINICAL PEARL

Start with a probiotic supplement that contains at least 3 billion CFUs, and consider gradually increasing the dose up to 45 billion CFUs as tolerated. Look for formulas that include *Lactobacillus* and *Bifidobacterium* strains. The most commonly studied species include *Lactobacillus acidophilus, Lactobacillus plantarum, Lactobacillus casei, Bifidobacterium breve, Bifidobacterium longum*, and *Bifidobacterium infantis*.

Probiotics can sometimes cause abdominal pain or bloating. If you do not tolerate them well or if they aren't helping to manage your diarrhea, it's perfectly okay to try another option.

Glutamine

L-Glutamine is an amino acid that supports immune function and promotes digestive health. During times of physical stress, illness, or injury, supplementation is necessary, which is why I use it as my go-to for persistent diarrhea after radiation treatment. Several clinical trials have demonstrated that glutamine is both safe and effective in reducing diarrhea in patients who have undergone pelvic radiation [16, 17].

CLINICAL PEARL

L-Glutamine is typically sold as a powder. The recommended daily dose is 5–15 g per day, for a minimum of one month. In many cases, diarrhea resolves completely; however, if your symptoms return, L-glutamine can also be taken on an as-needed basis.

Acupuncture

Another trusted approach I use for radiation-related diarrhea is acupuncture. It helps relax intestinal muscle contractions, easing pain and cramping. In my clinical experience, acupuncture provides effective and often lasting relief from diarrhea [18].

> **CLINICAL PEARL**
>
> Here is my go-to acupuncture protocol for diarrhea: SP6, ST36, ST37, SP9, SP15, ST25, LI4, LV3, SP3 and CV12. If available, apply a warming heat lamp over the abdomen during treatment. The sessions should be done twice weekly for 10–12 visits.

Side Effects of ADT

ADT is commonly prescribed when prostate cancer has spread beyond the prostate gland. This treatment lowers testosterone levels, which prostate cancer cells may depend on to grow. When testosterone drops, men can face significant physical and emotional changes. The most typical side effects include weight gain, muscle loss, hot flashes, depression, and anemia. Let's examine each of these and ways to manage them.

Complementary Therapies for Weight Gain

Within months of starting ADT, men may experience a significant increase in fat mass, up to 11% in the first year. Simultaneously, muscle mass may decrease by about 4% [19]. This shift in body composition can lead to increased cholesterol levels and higher blood sugar levels. It is starting to be recognized that men on ADT have a higher risk of developing diabetes, which can contribute to fatigue [20]. Additionally, men who gain weight during ADT are also at increased risk of developing cardiovascular disease compared to men who do not gain weight [21].

Changes in body shape can also affect self-esteem and overall quality of life. The best advice is to start preventive measures early. If you are about to start ADT, it's essential to be aware of the risk of weight gain and to maintain a balanced diet and regular exercise. Research shows that combining aerobic exercise, resistance training, and dietary counselling is an effective way to manage weight [22].

If you have already gained weight, Chapter 9 is dedicated to providing help with weight loss. If you have been diagnosed with diabetes and are feeling fatigued, Chapter 8 in this book focuses entirely on complementary therapies for managing diabetes. To prevent repeating content here, please refer to those chapters for a comprehensive review and a variety of complementary therapies to choose from.

Complementary Therapies for Hot Flashes

As discussed in the estrogen chapter, hot flashes are common when sex hormone levels decline. Up to 80% of men receiving ADT experience hot flashes [23]. These can be particularly disruptive at night, interrupting sleep, making it hard to fall back asleep, and resulting in fatigue.

Unfortunately, some treatments that work for women don't seem to be as effective in men. For example, soy and black cohosh have not shown consistent benefits in this group. The two I most often recommend for hot flashes in men are acupuncture and valerian root. Both have been proven to decrease the frequency and severity of hot flashes, helping men achieve more restful, uninterrupted sleep.

CLINICAL PEARL

Here is my acupuncture protocol for hot flashes: LV2, KI3, SP6, ST36, CV4, HT7, LI4, LI11, Shen men, and GV20.

CLINICAL PEARL

Dosing for valerian root varies among studies; however, I recommend starting with 300 mg in capsule form, taken three to four times daily (at breakfast, lunch, dinner, and before bed).

Complementary Therapies for Depression

Depending on the study, approximately one-third of men on ADT experience symptoms of depression [24]. The gold standard treatment is antidepressant therapy, but it is not without side effects and may not be very effective [25].

While some men may not receive a formal diagnosis of depression, it is very common for men with prostate cancer to have a low mood, which is also linked with low energy, poor sleep, poor appetite, and low self-worth [26]. Men with depression often don't report feelings of sadness or crying, as is frequently seen in women. Men typically describe feeling irritable, angry, or more hostile toward others, or experiencing problems with functioning at work. Other behaviors include aggressiveness, substance abuse, and escapism (over-involvement at work) [27].

Reasons for depression in men can include changes in body composition, a perceived lack of sexual prowess, poor sleep caused by hot flashes, low energy levels, and worries about the future. Men are less likely to seek help or talk to their doctors and loved ones about their feelings. If you are a man with prostate cancer reading this, remember you are not alone, and talking openly about how you feel is the first step toward coping and feeling better.

Depression is a vital symptom to address, so much so that Chapter 11 dedicates itself to complementary treatments for depression.

Complementary Therapies for Anemia

Testosterone plays a vital role in the production of red blood cells. When testosterone levels decrease, anemia can develop. Men undergoing ADT are roughly three times more likely to develop anemia than those not receiving this treatment. Hemoglobin, the protein in red blood cells that transports oxygen throughout the body, can decrease by up to 25%, leading to symptoms such as fatigue, shortness of breath, dizziness, and palpitations.

Iron deficiency is a common cause of anemia in men receiving ADT. Testosterone plays a role in nutrient absorption, and its absence can impair the body's ability to absorb iron as well as other key nutrients needed for blood cell production. In addition to iron deficiency, low levels of vitamin B12 and folate have also been found [28].

Anemia is essential to identify and treat, as it has been associated with a risk of cancer progression and lower survival times [29].

Once blood work confirms the presence of a nutrient deficiency, targeted supplementation can help restore hemoglobin levels and alleviate fatigue.

CLINICAL PEARL

For anemia caused by nutrient deficiency, consider the following supplementation plan: 5 mg of folic acid (preferably as 5-MTHF), 5,000 mcg of vitamin B12 via sublingual tablet, and 20 mg of elemental iron daily for three months. Reassess blood work at that time to evaluate the results.

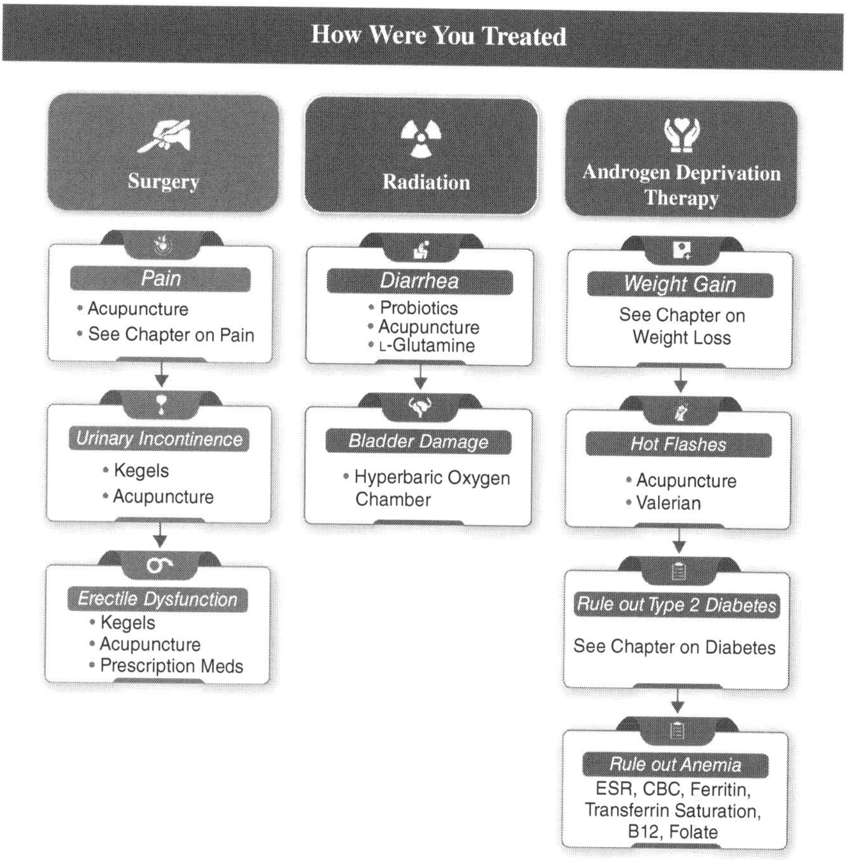

For Your Healthcare Practitioner

Clinicians should be especially vigilant when screening men on ADT for depression. A population-based study involving 180,189 men with prostate cancer revealed an increased risk of major depressive disorder (HR 1.82) and suicide (HR 2.43) [30]. Notably, this heightened risk persists for up to 10 years following diagnosis.

Particular attention should also be paid to racial disparities in mental health care. In a study of 78,313 men with prostate cancer treated with ADT, white men were three times more likely to be diagnosed with depression than Black men (30% vs. 10%). As a result, Black men were less likely to receive antidepressant therapy, underscoring the need for proactive screening and culturally sensitive care.

Iron deficiency anemia is often seen in men on ADT. The key mechanism is that low testosterone increases hepcidin, a liver-produced hormone that blocks iron absorption from the gut. Anemia of chronic disease is prevalent in this population, with one study reporting rates as high as 39.5%. This condition often presents with low serum iron and transferrin saturation (<20%), even when ferritin levels appear normal. When ruling out the cause of anemia, always ensure that you check transferrin saturation, ferritin, ESR, complete CBC, vitamin B12, and folate levels.

References

1 Luo YH, Yang YW, Wu CF, et al. Fatigue prevalence in men treated for prostate cancer: a systematic review and meta-analysis. World J Clin Cases, 2021; 9:5932–5942.
2 Gacci M, De Nunzio C, Sakalis V, et al. Latest evidence on post-prostatectomy urinary incontinence. J Clin Med, 2023; 12(3):1190.
3 Xiao J, Zhang M, Wu D. Side effects of prostate cancer therapies and potential management. J Biol Methods, 2024; 11(3):e99010018.
4 Ge TJ, Vetter J, Lai HH. Sleep disturbance and fatigue are associated with more severe urinary incontinence and overactive bladder symptoms. Urology, 2017; 109:67–73.
5 Konety BR, Sadetsky N, Carroll PR. Recovery of urinary continence following radical prostatectomy: the impact of prostate volume-analysis of data from the CaPSURE Database. J Urol, 2007; 177(4):1423–1425.
6 Yang Y, Rao C, Yin T, et al. Application and underlying mechanism of acupuncture for the nerve repair after peripheral nerve injury: remodelling of nerve system. Front Cell Neurosci, 2023; 17:1253438.
7 Walsh PC. The discovery of the cavernous nerves and development of nerve sparing radical retropubic prostatectomy. J Urol, 2007; 177(5):1632–1635.
8 Dorey G, Spearman M, Finely R, et al. Randomized controlled trial of pelvic floor muscle exercises and manometric biofeedback for erectile dysfunction. Br J Gen Pract, 2004; 54(508):819–825.
9 Pettersson N, Olsson C, Tucker SL, et al. Urethral pain among prostate cancer survivors 1 to 14 years after radiation therapy. Int J Radiat Oncol Biol Phys, 2013; 85(1):e29–e37.
10 Oscarsson N, Rosen A, Muller B, et al. Radiation-induced cystitis treated with hyperbaric oxygen therapy (RICH-ART): long-term follow-up of a randomized controlled, phase 2–3 study. EClinicalMedicine, 2025; 83:103214.
11 Fiorino C, Valdagni R, Rancati T, et al. Dose-volume effects for normal tissues in external radiotherapy. Pelvis Radiother Oncol 2009; 93(2):153–167.

12 Wang L, Wang X, Zhang G, et al. The impact of pelvic radiotherapy on the gut microbiome and its role in radiation-induced diarrhoea: a systematic review. Radiat Oncol, 2021; 16(1):187.

13 Artale S, Grillo N, Lepori S, et al. A nutritional approach for the management of chemotherapy-induced diarrhea in patients with colorectal cancer. Nutrients, 2022; 14(9):1801.

14 Delia P, Sansotta G, Donata V, et al. Probiotics for prevention of radiation-induced diarrhea. World J Gastroenterol, 2007; 13(6):912–915.

15 Khosroshahi RA, Zeraattalab-Motlagh S, Sarsangi P, et al. Effect of probiotic supplementation on chemotherapy- and radiotherarpy-related diarrhea in patients with cancer: an umbrella review of systematic reviews and meta-analysis. Br J Nutr, 2023; 130(10):1754–1765.

16 Peña Vivas JDC, Orduz Arena AC, Alonso García A, et al. Clinical, functional, and nutritional efficacy of a glutamine-enriched oligomeric diet in patients with rectal cancer. Nutr Cancer, 2024; 76(1):128–136.

17 Salas-Salas BG, Ferrera-Alayón L, Calleja-Fernández A, et al. Impact of a glutamine-enriched peptide formula on gastrointestinal toxicity and on the interruption of oncologic treatment in patients with adenocarcinoma of the rectum. Front Nutr, 2024; 11:1414367.

18 Wang Z, Hou Y, Sun H, et al. Efficacy of acupuncture treatment for diarrhea predominant irritable bowel syndrome with comorbid anxiety and depression: a meta-analysis and systematic review. Medicine (Baltimore), 2024; 103(46):e40207.

19 Pivonello R, Menafra D, Riccio E, et al. Metabolic disorders and male hypogonadotropic hypogonadism. Front Endocrinol (Lausanne), 2019; 10:345.

20 Saigal CS, Gore JL, Krupski TL, et al. Androgen deprivation therapy increases cardiovascular morbidity in men with prostate cancer. Cancer, 2007; 110(7):1493–1500.

21 Troeschel AN, Hartman TJ, Jacobs EJ, et al. Postdiagnosis body mass index, weight change, and mortality from prostate cancer, cardiovascular disease, and all causes among survivors of nonmetastatic prostate cancer. J Clin Oncol, 2020; 38:2018–2027.

22 Wilson RL, Taaffe DR, Newton RU, et al. Using exercise and nutrition to alter fat and lean mass in men with prostate cancer receiving androgen deprivation therapy: a narrative review. Nutrients, 2021; 13(5):1664.

23 Moyad MA, Complementary/alternative therapies for reducing hot flashes in prostate cancer patients: reevaluating the existing indirect data from studies from breast cancer and post menopausal women. Urology, 2002; 59(4):20–33.

24 Bassyouny NM, Gouda MM, Ezz El Din MM, et al. Impact of androgen deprivation therapy on cognitive function of elderly men with prostate cancer. Cureus, 2024; 16(9):e69303.

25 Alwhaibi A, Alsanea S, Almadi B, et al. Androgen deprivation therapy and depression in prostate cancer patients: review of risk and pharmacological management. Aging Male, 2022; 25(1):101–124.

26 Sharpley CF, Christie DRH, Arnold WM, et al. Network analysis of depression in prostate cancer patients: implications for assessment and treatment. Psychooncology, 2022; 32(3):368–374.

27 Cochran SV, Rabinowitz FE. Gender-sensitive recommendations for assessment and treatment of depression in men. Prof Psychol Res Pr, 2003; 34(2):132–140.

28 Wong CH, Ko I, Lee D, et al. Anemia and iron deficiency in advanced prostate cancer: revisiting a common morbidity. Hong Kong Med J, 2025; 31(2):154–158.

29 Caro JJ, Salas M, Ward A, et al. Anemia as an independent prognostic factor for survival in patients with cancer: a systemic, quantitative review. Cancer, 2001; 91:2214–2221.

30 Crump C, Stattin P, Brooks JD, et al. Long-term risks of depression and suicide among men with prostate cancer: a national cohort study. Eur Urol, 2023; 84(3):263–272.

Part III

Metabolic Changes

8

Tackling Diabetes Post Cancer

Anyone can give up; it is the easiest thing in the world to do. But to hold it together when everyone would expect you to fall apart, now that is true strength

—Chris Bradford

This chapter is for you if:

- You have been diagnosed with diabetes.
- You have had blood work that confirms you have prediabetes.
- You are feeling fatigued after cancer treatment, and you are wondering about insulin resistance.

Uncovering the root cause of your fatigue often requires some detective work, and diabetes is a stealthy culprit that can be surprisingly easy to overlook. Diabetes is a condition that impacts how our bodies manage blood sugar, with the most common type being type 2 diabetes (T2DM). T2DM is a major health concern worldwide, and its prevalence is continuing to rise [1]. It's marked by having too much sugar in the blood (hyperglycemia). When blood sugar levels are poorly controlled, it can lead to a range of health issues, including fatigue.

So, why does diabetes cause fatigue? Mainly because your body can't effectively use sugar for energy. When your blood sugar is high, there's plenty of fuel in your bloodstream, but it can't easily enter your cells where it's needed. This occurs because the body isn't producing enough insulin (the hormone that helps sugar enter cells), or your cells are no longer responding to it (called insulin resistance). So, even with enough "fuel" present, your cells—your body's energy factories—aren't getting what they need, which leads to that tired feeling.

But that's just part of the story. When blood sugar is high, your kidneys have to work extra hard to eliminate it, leading to increased urination and fluid loss. This can leave you feeling dehydrated, which adds to your fatigue. Additionally,

Beyond Cancer Fatigue: A Path to Reclaiming Energy, First Edition. Jessa Landmann, ND.

a common diabetes medication called metformin can sometimes reduce your vitamin B12 levels, which might cause anemia and tiredness [2].

The relationship between diabetes and cancer is complex. We're learning that people who have T2DM have a higher risk of developing certain types of cancers, including breast and prostate cancer [3]. On the flip side, some cancer treatments themselves can unfortunately raise the risk of developing diabetes in survivors of leukemia, as well as cancers of the breast, prostate, colon, head and neck, and pancreas [4].

The impact of diabetes in people with cancer stretches far beyond numbers on a lab report. They face a higher risk of more severe side effects from cancer treatments, such as infections, drops in white blood cell counts, and neuropathy [5]. Cancer survivors with diabetes are also at higher risk of anxiety, depression, pain, and low overall physical functioning [6]. And very importantly, high blood sugar has been linked to poorer overall survival and a higher risk of cancer recurrence [7].

This all underscores the vital importance of identifying and managing diabetes, especially for cancer survivors. Here's the key takeaway: controlling your blood sugar is not just important for diabetes itself, but it can also significantly impact how you feel during and after cancer treatment. By addressing diabetes, you can lessen fatigue and improve your overall health and wellness.

Cancer Drugs That May Cause Diabetes

Undergoing cancer treatment can raise the risk of diabetes for some individuals. If you've received any of the treatments listed below, you should undergo a comprehensive assessment for diabetes and insulin resistance.

a. Chemotherapy—High blood sugar occurs in about 10–30% of people receiving chemotherapy. While often temporary, it can sometimes become chronic and eventually lead to a diagnosis of diabetes. Some common chemotherapy drugs linked to this include 5-fluorouracil (5-FU), platinum agents (cisplatin, carboplatin, oxaliplatin), and anthracyclines (doxorubicin, epirubicin) [8].

b. Targeted agents—These are newer drugs with significant potential for cancer control, but some, like the drug Everolimus [9], increase the risk of diabetes.

c. Androgen deprivation therapy (ADT)—This is a treatment for men with prostate cancer, and has been strongly linked with an increased risk of diabetes [10].

d. Tamoxifen—One of the most commonly used drugs on the market is an anti-estrogen medication used for treating hormone-positive breast cancer, and rates of diabetes in these women may be as high as 10% [11].

e. Steroids—The use of steroid medications, such as dexamethasone and prednisone, is common during chemotherapy to reduce swelling, relieve pain, reduce nausea, or boost appetite. Blood sugar increases almost immediately after ingestion of steroid drugs, and about 1 in 10 people treated with steroids will develop diabetes [12].

Diabetes Screening and Assessment

Let's now review the blood tests used to evaluate diabetes and their optimal values:

	Healthy	Prediabetes	Diabetes
Fasting blood sugar	Less than 6 mmol/L	Between 6.1–6.9 mmol/L	Greater than 7 mmol/L
Random blood sugar	Between 3.5–7 mmol/L	Between 7–11 mmol/L	Greater than 11.1 mmol/L
HbA1C	Less than 5.7%	Between 5.7–6.4%	Greater than 6.5%

Identifying and managing prediabetes is essential because it is strongly linked to the development of full-blown T2DM and cardiovascular disease [13]. If left untreated, 5–10% of individuals with prediabetes may develop T2DM each year [14].

To detect prediabetes, in addition to blood sugar levels mentioned above, you should ask your doctor to perform the HOMA-IR score. HOMA-IR stands for Homeostatic Model Assessment of Insulin Resistance, and it measures insulin resistance.

Insulin resistance is a condition that occurs before diabetes, in which the body's cells do not respond well to the hormone insulin, which carries sugar into the cells. This leads to fatigue because your cells aren't receiving the energy they need.

To calculate this, you should request a fasting insulin and fasting glucose blood test from your doctor. You can then easily enter those values into an online HOMA-IR calculator to obtain your score. Generally, a score below 1.0 is ideal, while anything above 2.5 indicates the need for attention and potential treatment.

CLINICAL PEARL

One of the early signs and symptoms that might indicate prediabetes is muscle fatigue. A common complaint I hear from people recovering from cancer treatments, even those with ample muscle mass, is feeling tired and experiencing weak muscles. Activities like walking, climbing stairs, or even daily tasks can become exhausting. If you notice tired muscles, especially in the legs, it is important to be evaluated for prediabetes and to calculate your HOMA-IR score.

REFLECTION POINT

Take a moment to review the cancer treatments you've received in the past and consider whether you might be at risk of diabetes. Also, ask yourself if you've been regularly checking your blood sugar with a finger-prick test. If not, when was the last time you had a comprehensive blood sugar panel done? Do you experience muscular fatigue? All of these could be reasons to screen for insulin resistance and diabetes, especially if you continue to feel fatigued.

Complementary Treatments for Diabetes

Exercise Programming for Diabetes

Exercise has been proven to lower blood sugar levels and decrease the risk of diabetes. Both aerobic exercise and weight lifting are beneficial, and combining them provides the greatest benefits for blood sugar control. Aerobic exercise boosts the rate at which sugar is cleared from the blood because your body requires more energy, while resistance training builds muscle, which is a key organ involved in removing sugar from the blood [15].

Maintaining high muscle mass has long been recognized as a protective factor against diabetes and prediabetes [16]. In particular, growing the muscles in the lower limbs (glutes, hamstrings, quadriceps) is essential and should be the focus of resistance training [17]. These muscles are some of the largest in the body and are rich in mitochondria. The more muscle and mitochondria we have, the more fuel is burned, which helps lower blood sugar levels and reduce fat [18].

What is exciting and very encouraging is that it matters less what kind of exercise you do, but more about the time you spend. A fascinating study looked at different exercise regimens in people with prediabetes and diabetes. They discovered that while combined aerobic and resistance exercise was more effective in lowering blood sugar than either type of exercise alone, the difference was not statistically significant. What seemed to be most important was the time spent exercising, and they came up with some guidelines below [19]:

Type of exercise	Intensity	Minimum amount	Ideal amount
Aerobic exercise only	Moderate	3 days per week, 25 minutes each or 5 days per week, 15 minutes each	3 days per week, 65 minutes each or 5 days per week, 40 minutes each
	Vigorous	3 days per week, 15 minutes each or 5 days per week, 10 minutes each	3 days per week, 35 minutes each or 5 days per week, 20 minutes each
Resistance training only	Moderate	3 days per week, 25 minutes each or 5 days per week, 15 minutes each	3 days per week, 60 minutes each or 5 days per week, 35 minutes each
	Vigorous	3 days per week, 15 minutes each or 5 days per week, 10 minutes each	3 days per week, 40 minutes each or 5 days per week, 25 minutes each
Combined aerobic and resistance exercise	Moderate	3 days per week, 45 minutes each or 5 days per week, 25 minutes each	3 days per week, 55 minutes each or 5 days per week, 30 minutes each

If you haven't been exercising for a while, start with the guidelines in the minimum amount column. These are very achievable goals. The minimum recommended amount of aerobic exercise is just 15 minutes daily, five days a week. As you build a habit and gain momentum, you can gradually work your way up to the targets in the ideal amount column. While the primary goal of this exercise program is to lower blood sugar, bcing more active and building muscle will also significantly boost your energy levels.

For some inspiration, here is a list of activities classified as moderate or vigorous in intensity. Choose something you enjoy and follow the time guidelines from the table above to get started.

MODERATE LEVEL ACTIVITIES	
Dancing	Jumping on a mini trampoline
Badminton	Kayaking
Baseball	Raking leaves
Shooting hoops	Shoveling snow
Leisurely biking	Downhill skiing
Brisk walking	Slow swimming
Gardening	Tennis
Ice skating	Volleyball

VIGOROUS LEVEL ACTIVITIES	
Vigorous basketball game	Rollerblading
Biking 20 km/hour	Soccer
Touch football	Fast swimming
Ultimate frisbee	Speed walking
Hockey	Climbing stairs
Jogging or running	Water polo
Racquetball	Cross-country skiing
Hiking	Jumping rope

A Note on Light Exercise and Reducing Sedentary Behavior

If moderate- or vigorous-level exercise feels out of reach, light exercise can also help lower blood sugar. Studies have looked at gentle forms of movement, such as chair yoga or Tai chi, and found that even these types of activities can lower blood sugar [20].

Even just standing more often and reducing sedentariness can lower blood sugar and improve your health. Older or frail individuals often spend a significant amount of their time sitting. Modern society has created a lifestyle where people of all ages spend a substantial portion of their day sitting. From students to daily commuters and remote workers who've turned their kitchens into offices, many of us spend far too much time sitting

Sitting for long periods is now recognized as a significant risk factor for developing type 2 diabetes and can also increase the risk of death from any cause [21]. Even those who exercise regularly should avoid prolonged sedentary behavior, as sitting for extended periods has been linked to the development of illness, regardless of regular physical activity [22].

If you're having trouble with blood sugar control, even light physical activity can make a difference. Taking a short walk after a meal or simply standing and doing some light tidying can help lower your blood sugar levels [23]. Switching from a seated to a standing position throughout the day can boost your calorie burn, elevate your heart rate, and lower your blood sugar levels [24].

CLINICAL PEARL

If your day consists of significant sitting time, set a reminder every 20 minutes to get up and walk around, or set a timer to alternate between sitting and standing every 20 minutes, especially for the two hours after you eat.

REFLECTION POINT

Begin to track your daily routine and be aware of how much time you spend sitting or reclining. Do you spend a lot of time driving? Look for opportunities throughout your day to get up and move around. From the list above, take a moment to consider the activities you enjoy or new ones you might like to try. Where in your day can you fit in this activity?

Nutrition Interventions for Diabetes

Poor nutrition is a key factor contributing to T2DM, so it makes sense that improving your eating habits will directly improve diabetes control. With knowledge, commitment, and effort, you can significantly boost your energy and substantially improve your long-term health outlook.

Nutrition for Prediabetes

People with prediabetes are very prone to gaining weight. These individuals should limit their intake of foods that cause rapid increases in blood sugar, such as white rice, white bread, white potatoes, sugary drinks, processed foods, and baked goods. Instead, they should concentrate on whole grains and high-fiber foods such as leafy greens, sweet potatoes, berries, lentils, beans, oats, brown rice, and whole-grain breads. Prediabetics often see the most significant weight loss with this dietary approach [25].

Nutrition for Diabetics

There has been considerable debate in the field of nutrition research about the best dietary approach for individuals with diabetes. Very low-calorie diets have been studied, which have been shown to lead to weight loss and improved blood sugar control. However, the main challenge with calorie restriction is its lack of long-term sustainability and the high risk of regaining weight.

Low-carbohydrate diets have also been studied, with some success in achieving weight loss and blood sugar control. However, limiting carbohydrates may limit fiber content, and it is also difficult to sustain long-term, with a high risk of weight regain [26].

As you've read elsewhere throughout the writing on these pages, this book emphasizes adopting eating patterns that are non-restrictive, sustainable, enjoyable, nourishing, healthy, and, most importantly, delicious. Labeling your diet as being "low-calorie" or "low carb" may create a restrictive feeling and hinder long-term success.

High-sugar foods and refined carbohydrates (white rice, white bread, processed foods) are the biggest threat to those with diabetes, and avoidance of these foods is critical. Mediterranean diets [27] and ketogenic diets [28] have both been shown to lower blood sugar and lead to weight loss. In Chapter 9, covering weight loss, a more detailed breakdown of each of these eating patterns will be provided.

A ketogenic diet and a Mediterranean diet share many similarities. If you examine the food pyramids in the following chapter, you'll notice that the ketogenic diet emphasizes healthy fats more. Both dietary patterns limit refined grains (such as white breads) and other high-sugar foods, while promoting fiber intake through fruits and vegetables.

One notable fiber source is ground flaxseed. Flaxseed is rich in healthy fats, and ample research supports its beneficial role in health and disease, particularly in cardiovascular health. It has been shown to lower blood pressure, lower cholesterol, and lower blood sugar [29]. Flaxseed helps prevent or slow the absorption of sugars into the body, which is beneficial for people with diabetes [30].

Since it is well known that sticking to any specific "diet" long-term often leads to dropouts and relapses, it might be beneficial to switch between different eating patterns. One study that alternated between a ketogenic diet and a Mediterranean diet found that long-term adherence was high, resulting in significant weight loss and reduced blood sugar levels over a year [31].

CLINICAL PEARL

The Mediterranean diet is an excellent option for managing diabetes through proper nutrition. Make sure to include 1–2 tablespoons of ground flax in your daily intake of healthy fats.

Success Story

Jorge was a cancer survivor who overcame stage III colon cancer. He visited me two years after his diagnosis with a chief complaint of fatigue. Before his diagnosis, he had managed diabetes for 10 years, and the only medication he took was metformin. He was not informed that metformin could decrease vitamin B12 levels, nor had he ever taken it as a supplement. Over the past two years, since his surgery, he had become increasingly tired, unable to even go for walks, and had gained about 15 pounds.

We checked his HbA1C, which was 7.1%. His vitamin B12 level was 206. When reviewing his daily nutritional intake, he admitted to having a low appetite due to depression and reported eating only one meal per day.

We discussed how a high-protein diet (chicken, turkey, salmon, trout) could increase energy levels, boost vitamin B12 levels, and lower blood sugar. High-protein diets can enhance feelings of fullness and help replace carbohydrate-rich foods, thereby promoting a healthier diet. His goal was 140 g of protein daily.

To give him a boost, I administered an intramuscular injection of vitamin B12. He reported feeling more energetic afterward and began exercising for 20 minutes per day on his exercise bike. We discussed how increased muscle mass in the lower leg could significantly help lower blood sugar, and he felt this was an achievable exercise goal.

After three months, we retested his blood work, which showed that his HbA1C levels had dropped to 5.6%, his vitamin B12 levels had increased to 495, he had lost 13 pounds, and his mood and energy had substantially improved.

Fatty Liver

One of the most common features of T2DM is fatty liver disease, which is caused by the accumulation of excess fat, sugar, and insulin in the body. It is estimated that about 50–75% of diabetics have fatty liver [32]. Not only does fatty liver perpetuate diabetes, but it can also cause other serious health consequences, such as liver cirrhosis or liver cancer [33]. Treating fatty liver can improve diabetes control [34] and increase your energy.

Several effective eating habits have been studied. First, a high protein intake reduces fat deposits in the liver. Consuming high-protein foods helps you lose weight, replaces other high-fat and high-sugar foods, and may stimulate genes that promote fat breakdown in both the liver and abdomen [35]. However, the type of protein matters: choose lean, unprocessed options like fish, poultry, tofu, legumes, and eggs.

Second, the Mediterranean diet is also effective for fatty liver disease, particularly when carbohydrates (such as bread, pasta, and grains) are limited and a focus is placed on healthy fats and lean proteins [36]. Carbohydrates from fruits and vegetables are encouraged, as these foods are anti-inflammatory and can help support liver and metabolic health.

While lifestyle changes, such as a healthy diet and exercise, should always be the cornerstone of fatty liver treatment, one particular supplement stands out as a helpful adjunct. Curcumin is an extract from the root of the turmeric plant, and it possesses strong anti-inflammatory properties. Extensive research supports the recommendation that curcumin is effective in reducing liver fat, inhibiting liver fibrosis, and enhancing liver function [37].

CLINICAL PEARL

Curcumin, when combined with other lifestyle modifications, is efficacious in improving fatty liver disease. The dose in clinical trials ranges from 250 to 500 mg per day.

Supplements for Diabetes

Proper nutrition and regular exercise should always form the foundation for managing diabetes. They not only help control blood sugar and support weight management but also energize our bodies through physical activity and a balanced diet of healthy foods. When blood sugar cannot be kept in check with diet and exercise alone, prescription medications will be necessary. These are essential drugs, and if advised by your doctor, you should always follow their guidance.

Several supplements can also help lower blood sugar and support overall metabolic health. Supplements shouldn't replace prescription medication, but they may be a helpful add-on to your care.

Berberine

Berberine is present in various medicinal plants that have been used for thousands of years to treat ailments such as allergies, infections, and arthritis. It has also been found to be valuable in lowering blood sugar and cholesterol, reducing fatty liver, and aiding weight loss [38].

In one clinical trial, berberine was found to be as effective as metformin in controlling blood sugar levels [39]. Berberine can also be used together with metformin in people who, despite being on medication, are still having difficulty managing their sugar levels [40]. It can also be effectively used in people with prediabetes [41].

CLINICAL PEARL

Berberine is an over-the-counter supplement that can be taken safely to help regulate blood sugar levels and improve energy. Start with a dose of 500 mg twice daily, but this can be increased to 1,000 mg twice daily if needed. Monitor blood work at least every three months to ensure you are getting the results you need.

Success Story

Bernadette was a 76-year-old woman who had battled ovarian cancer for 10 years. She admitted to having low motivation to eat properly or to exercise. She had a rich family life, with two daughters, four grandchildren, and a loving husband.

Over the past two years, her fasting blood sugar and HbA1C gradually increased, and she noticed her energy levels steadily dropping. We discussed lifestyle changes, but she was resistant. I recommended berberine to help lower her blood sugar and explained that it would boost her energy and benefit her overall health. After one month of taking berberine, her fasting blood sugar dropped from 13.6 to 6.8. She felt more energetic to play with her grandchildren and manage her day-to-day activities.

Cinnamon

You might already enjoy cinnamon as a comforting addition to your breakfast or baking, but perhaps you didn't know you can also find it in supplement form over the counter. Similar to berberine, it lowers blood sugar in diabetics and pre-diabetics [42], and reduces cholesterol levels as well [43].

CLINICAL PEARL

Cinnamon supplement, at doses of 3–4 g per day, can help improve blood sugar levels and, as a result, boost energy levels.

Bitter Melon

Bitter melon is a unique tropical fruit commonly found in many parts of Asia, rich in vitamins and minerals. One of its most notable qualities is its ability to lower blood sugar levels. It lowers HbA1C, fasting glucose [44], and may help with weight loss, reduce body fat, and lower waist circumference [45].

You can lower blood sugar by eating the fruit; however, its bitter taste and limited availability in many grocery stores make it a less appealing choice for some. It is available in supplement form, and because the doses can be more precise in pill form, this is the recommended way to take bitter melon for blood sugar.

CLINICAL PEARL

Doses in clinical trials range from 300 mg to 2,000 mg per day. I suggest starting with 1,000 mg daily for three months and monitoring your blood sugar to assess its effectiveness. If, after three months, no clear benefits are shown, increase the dose to 1,500 mg, then to 2,000 mg.

Conclusion

Given the intricate link between cancer survivorship and an elevated risk of diabetes, understanding and addressing this connection is paramount. Diabetes not only intensifies cancer-related fatigue but also introduces a cascade of other health complications. Therefore, proactive assessment of prediabetes and diabetes, coupled with diligent blood sugar management, isn't just about preventing further health issues, but flourishing as the healthiest version of you.

References

1 International Diabetes Federation. IDF Diabetes Atlas 2021. Available at https://diabetesatlas.org/atlas/tenth-edition/.
2 Sayedali E, Yalin AE, Yalin S. Association between metformin and vitamin B12 deficiency in patients with type 2 diabetes. World J Diabetes, 2023; 14(5):585–593.
3 Gong Z, Neuhouser ML, Goodmas PJ, et al. Obesity, diabetes and risk of prostate cancer: results from the prostate cancer prevention trial. Cancer Epidemiol Biomarkers Prev, 2006; 15(10):1977.
4 Jo A, Scarton L, O'Neal LJ, et al. New onset of type 2 diabetes as a complication after cancer diagnosis: a systematic review. Cancer Med, 2021; 10:439–446.
5 Alenzi EO, Kelley GA. The association of hyperglycemia and diabetes mellitus and the risk of chemotherapy induced neutropenia among cancer patients: a systemic review with meta-analysis. J Diabetes Complications, 2017; 31(1):267–272.
6 Ose DJ, Adediran E, Mark B, et al. The association of diabetes and routinely collected patient reported outcomes in patients with cancer: a real world cohort study. Cancer Med, 2024; 13:e70246.
7 Bar R, Templeton AJ, Seruga B, et al. Hyperglycemia and survival in solid tumours: a systematic review and meta-analysis. Clin Oncol, 2018; 30(4):215–224.
8 Teng CJ, Chang KH, Tsai IJ, et al. Impact of anthracycline on diabetes mellitus development in B-cell lymphoma patients: a nationwide population-based study. Clin Drug Investig, 2018; 38(7):603–610.
9 Verges B. mTOR and cardiovascular diseases: diabetes mellitus. Transplantation, 2018; 102(2):S47–S49.
10 Keating NL, O'Malley A, Freedland SJ, et al. Diabetes and cardiovascular disease during androgen deprivation therapy: observational study of veterans with prostate cancer. J Natl Cancer Inst, 2012; 104(19):1518–1523.

11 Lipscombe LL, Fischer HD, Yun L, et al. Association between tamoxifen treatment and diabetes: a population-based study. Cancer, 2012; 118(10):2615–2622.

12 Pilkey J, Streeter L, Beel A, et al. Corticosteroid-induced diabetes in palliative care. J Palliat Med, 2012; 15(6):681–689.

13 Yi J, Qu C, Li X. Insulin resistance assessed by estimated glucose disposal rate and risk of atherosclerotic cardiovascular diseases incidence: the multi-ethnic study of atherosclerosis. Cardiovasc Diabetol, 2024; 23(1):349.

14 Menke A, Casagrande S, Geiss L, et al. Prevalence of and trends in diabetes among adults in the United States, 1988–2012. JAMA, 2015; 314:1021–1029.

15 Kanaley JA, Colberg SR, Corcoran MH, et al. Exercise/physical activity in individuals with type 2 diabetes: a consensus statement from the American College of Sports Medicine. Med Sci Sports Exerc, 2022; 54:353–368.

16 Srikanthan P, Karlamangla AS. Relative muscle mass is inversely associated with insulin resistance and prediabetes. Findings from the third national health and nutrition survey. J Clin Endocr Metab, 2011; 96(9):2898–2903.

17 Seko T, Akasaka H, Koyama M, et al. Preserved lower limb muscle mass prevents insulin resistance development in non-diabetic older adults. J Am Med Direct Assoc, 2023; 24(3):376–381.

18 Fukushima Y, Kurose S, Shinno H, et al. Importance of lean muscle maintenance to improve insulin resistance by body weight reduction in female patients with obesity. Diabetes Metab J, 2016; 40:147–153.

19 Zhang L, Cheng X, Yang Y, et al. Optimal dosage and modality of exercise on glycemic control in people with prediabetes: a systematic review and network meta-analysis. Endocrinol (Lausanne), 2025; 16:1560676.

20 Zhao W, Ju H, Zhu K. Meta-analysis of the intervention effects of tai chi on fasting blood glucose, blood pressure and triglyceride in middle-aged and elderly people. Aging Male, 2024; 27(1):2282977.

21 Gao W, Sanna M, Chen Y, et al. Occupational sitting time, leisure physical activity, and all-cause and cardiovascular disease mortality. JAMA Netw Open, 2024; 7(1):e2350680.

22 Peter TK, Timothy SC, Cora LC, et al. Sitting time and mortality from all causes, cardiovascular disease, and cancer. Med Sci Sports Exerc, 2009; 41:998–1005.

23 Chinmay M, James AI, Debashis KN, et al. The effect of walking on postprandial glycemic excursion in patients with type 1 diabetes and healthy people. Diabetes Care, 2012; 35:2493–2499.

24 Dobashi S, Kawaguchi S, Ando D, et al. Alternating work posture improves postprandial glucose response without reducing computer task performance in the early afternoon. Physiol Behav, 2021; 237:113431.

25 Hjorth MF, Ritz C, Blaak EE, et al. Pretreatment fasting plasma glucose and insulin modify dietary weight loss success: results from 3 randomized clinical trials. Am J Clin Nutr, 2017; 106:499–505.
26 Taylor R, Ramachandran A, Yancy WS, et al. Nutritional basis of type 2 diabetes remission. BMJ, 2021; 374:n1449.
27 Huo R, Du T, Xu Y, et al. Effects of mediterranean-style diet on glycemic control, weight loss and cardiovascular risk factors among type 2 diabetes individuals: a meta-analysis. Eur J Clin Nutr, 2015; 69:1200–1208.
28 Zhou C, Wang M, Liang J, et al. Ketogenic diet benefits to weight loss, glycemic control, and lipid profiles in overweight patients with type 2 diabetes mellitus: a meta-analysis of randomized controlled trials. Int J Environ Res Public Health, 2022; 19:10429.
29 Kunutsor SK, Jassal DS, Ravandi A, et al. Dietary flaxseed: cardiometabolic benefits and its role in promoting healthy aging. Geroscience, 2025; 47(3):2895–2923.
30 López-Toledo S, Pineda De la Cruz MC, Gutiérrez-Hurtado IA, et al. Flaxseed improves glucose and lipid metabolism in Mexican subjects with type 2 diabetes: a parallel randomized clinical trial. Nutrients, 2025; 17(4):709.
31 Paoli A, Bianco A, Grimaldi KA, et al. Long term successful weight loss with a combination biphasic ketogenic Mediterranean diet and Mediterranean diet maintenance protocol. Nutrients, 2013; 5:5205–5217.
32 Gupte P, Amarapurkar D, Agal S, et al. Non-alcoholic steatohepatitis in type 2 diabetes mellitus. J Gastroenterol Hepatol, 2004; 19:854–858.
33 Tolman KG, Fonseca V, Tan MH, et al. A narrative review: hepatobiliary disease in type 2 diabetes mellitus. Ann Intern Med, 2004; 141:946–956.
34 Lim EL, Hollingsworth KG, Aribisala BS, et al. Reversal of type 2 diabetes: normalisation of beta cell function in association with decreased pancreas and liver triacylglycerol. Diabetologia, 2011; 54:2506–2514.
35 Bortolotti M, Kreis R, Debard C, et al. High protein intake reduces intrahepatocellular lipid deposition in humans. Am J Clin Nutr, 2009; 90:1002–1010.
36 Haigh L, Kirk C, Gendy KE, et al. The effectiveness and acceptability of mediterranean diet and calorie restriction in non-alcoholic fatty liver disease (NAFLD): a systematic review and meta-analysis. Clin Nutr, 2022; 41(9):1913–1931.
37 Handu D, Stote K, Piemonte T. Evaluating bioactive-substance-based interventions for adults with MASLD: results from a systematic scoping review. Nutrients, 2025; 17(3):453.
38 Ilyas Z, Perna S, Al-Thawadi S, et al. The effect of berberine on weight loss in order to prevent obesity: a systematic review. Biomed Pharmacother, 2020; 127:110137.

39 Yin J, Xing H, Ye J. Efficacy of berberine in patients with type 2 diabetes. Metabolism, 2008; 57(5):712–717.

40 Sartore G, Ragazzi E, Antonello G, et al. Effect of a new formulation of nutraceuticals as add-on to metformin mono therapy for patients with type 2 diabetes and suboptimal glycemic control: a randomized controlled trial. Nutrients, 2021; 13(7):2373.

41 Panigrahi A, Mohanty S. Efficacy and safety of HIMABERB Berberine on glycemic control in patients with prediabetes: a double-blind, placebo-controlled, and randomized pilot trial. BMC Endocr Discord, 2023; 23(1):190.

42 Zelicha H, Yang J, Henning SM, et al. Effect of cinnamon spice on continuously monitored glycemic response in adult with prediabetes: a 4-week randomized controlled crossover trial. Am J Clin Nutr, 2024; 119(3):649–657.

43 Lira Neto JCG, Araújo MFM, Araújo AVEC, et al. Effectiveness of cinnamon in the reduction of lipid levels in people with diabetes: a randomized clinical trial. Rev Gaucha Enferm, 2023; 44:e20230051.

44 Mes JJ, van den Belt M, van der Haar S, et al. Bitter gourd (*Momordica charantia* L.) supplementation for twelve weeks improves biomarkers of glucose homeostasis in a prediabetic population. J Ethnopharmacol, 2025; 347:119756.

45 Cortez-Navarrete M, Martínez-Abundis E, Pérez-Rubio KG, et al. Momordica charantia administration improves insulin secretion in type 2 diabetes mellitus. J Med Food, 2018; 21(7):672–677.

9

Peace with Food, Power with Weight Loss

If you want to accomplish anything in life, you can't just sit back and hope it will happen. You've got to make it happen

—Chuck Norris

What I know for sure is this: The big secret in life is that there is no secret. Whatever your goal for this year is, you can get there, as long as you're willing to be honest with yourself about the preparation and work involved. There are no back doors, no free rides. There's just you, this moment, and a choice

—Oprah

This chapter is for you if:

- You have experienced weight gain since starting cancer treatment.
- You have previously tried to lose weight without success and are now seeking a new approach.
- You struggle with emotional eating and want to develop a healthier relationship with food.

Let's begin this chapter by taking a few deep breaths. Weight can be a very personal issue, and it's essential to approach this topic with kindness and understanding toward ourselves. Maybe you've always carried some extra weight, or perhaps you've noticed your weight creep up during your cancer treatment and recovery. Please remember that this is a common experience, and you're not alone.

This chapter isn't about chasing an ideal body or feeling shame about where you are right now. Instead, it's about exploring how gently shifting toward a healthy weight can increase your energy, enhance your overall well-being, and support your long-term health. Please think of this chapter as part of a journey

Beyond Cancer Fatigue: A Path to Reclaiming Energy, First Edition. Jessa Landmann, ND.

of self-care, where we'll explore practical and sustainable ways to nourish both your body and mind.

In Hale Sofia Schatz's book, "If the Buddha Came to Dinner," the author asks a compelling question: What would you feed Buddha, this spiritual being, if he came to your home for a meal? Would you serve him fast food or a microwave meal? Or would you want to prepare a beautiful dinner, made from scratch, with colors and delicious flavors?

The author then asks, what would you feed another spiritual being—yourself! The book challenges you to see yourself as a special being who is also deserving of wonderful meals. She encourages nourishing yourself with intention, beauty, and care, with the same respect you would give to an honored guest.

The book promotes mindful eating by encouraging you to pay attention to what's on your plate, enjoy the aroma and flavor of your food, and learn to listen to your body's hunger and fullness cues. Its central message is to turn eating into a daily practice that nourishes both body and mind, redefining our relationship with food and moving away from calorie counting as a weight-loss strategy. The focus is on building awareness, which facilitates intentional choices that, in turn, lead to actions. It's these actions that generate long-term, sustainable results.

Why Have We Gained Weight in the First Place

You've read in earlier chapters about factors related to cancer and its treatment that can lead to weight gain. Hormone-blocking agents used for treating breast and prostate cancer cause changes in metabolism and disrupt sleep. Mental and emotional factors, such as stress and depression, may also interfere with sleep or decrease motivation to exercise. Cancer often creates a perfect storm of changes that contribute to struggles with weight.

However, cancer aside, obesity is a modern-day issue. While it's not exactly clear when the "modern day" began, it is generally believed that the obesity epidemic started in Westernized nations between 1976 and 1980 [1]. Obesity is now recognized as a global epidemic, as what was once seen as a problem of Westernized countries due to an excess of food, emerging markets now have access to "fast food" and are also struggling with obesity.

It's also now the leading risk factor for developing cancer, surpassing cigarettes. That may be a surprising fact. Most people are aware that cigarettes cause lung cancer and cancers of the mouth and throat. But many are unaware of the adverse health effects of the foods they eat and the drinks they consume. The obesity epidemic has largely been blamed on the availability of soda drinks and ultra-processed foods [2].

Many books describe how food manufacturers carefully manipulate taste and texture to attract consumers. If you're interested in learning more, consider

Michael Moss's books, "Salt, Sugar, Fat: How the Food Giants Hooked Us" and "Hooked: Food, Free Will, and How the Food Giants Exploit our Addiction."

Research confirms that ultra-processed foods can be addictive. They are high in salt, sugar, fat, and chemical ingredients, and lack significant nutritional value. These foods are designed to send quick signals to the brain, stimulating pleasure centers and releasing dopamine rapidly. When dopamine activates the brain's reward system, it can lead to addiction.

These foods not only contribute to weight gain but also raise the risk of cardiovascular disease and diabetes. People who consume a lot of ultra-processed foods tend to have poorer sleep and higher levels of depression and anxiety [3]. Over time, they leave us feeling tired and drained.

Emotional eating contributes to obesity, as our feelings can cause us to make unhealthy food choices and consume excess food. Cancer survivors coping with stress or sadness might turn to food for comfort and distraction. Emotional eating often overrides the body's natural hunger signals, making us unaware of the brain's cues for hunger or fullness.

Time scarcity is a common complaint in our modern world, and many feel they don't have time to cook. Some people may work long hours or have many responsibilities that cause food preparation to take a back seat; as a result, fast food becomes the easier choice. By recognizing these barriers, we can begin to identify what's blocking healthier choices and what small changes might help.

REFLECTION POINT

In your journal, write down any concepts you've identified that may be contributing to weight gain or difficulty losing weight. Do you eat processed foods often and worry you might be addicted? Do you notice that you eat more when stressed or sad? Are you busy driving your kids to activities, making it hard to prepare dinner, and leading you to eat out at fast-food restaurants? Be gentle and curious. Jot down a few thoughts that come to mind. No judgment, just awareness.

Weight Loss Methods

Step 1: Ensure Your Metabolism is Working

Many believe that eating less helps with weight loss, but extreme restriction can actually lower your metabolic rate. The basal metabolic rate (BMR) is the number of calories required for basic functions, such as breathing and blood flow.

Here's what you need to know: the higher your BMR, the easier it is to lose weight. Factors that increase your BMR include having more muscle mass and eating enough food. Weight lifting at least two to three days per week is highly recommended. Conversely, factors that lower BMR include prolonged inactivity and under-eating.

How can you determine your BMR? You can use a free online BMR calculator at www.calculator.net. Enter your age, height, and weight, and it will calculate your BMR. Keep in mind that your daily calorie needs will vary depending on your level of activity.

Once you have calculated your BMR, aim to eat at least that number of calories daily. To fully understand how many calories you are consuming, it is strongly recommended that you track your food intake. Tracking your intake is essential to stay on track, so you can feel certain that you are taking in enough calories, but not more than you need.

The most convenient way to track your food intake is with a smartphone app. One popular and easy-to-use app is MyFitnessPal, which enables you to record exactly what you eat. It not only monitors your calories but also your protein, carbohydrate, and fat intake. Other popular apps include Chronometer, Lifesum, and Lose It. All of them are free, so take a look and choose the one that best suits you.

How you get in those calories matters, though. Let's say your BMR is 1,500. It's not ideal to hit that target with burgers and fries. Below is a list of allowable foods to give you a guide. Once you have calculated your BMR, you can eat whatever you want from the food list below, provided you track your food intake to ensure you don't exceed your daily limit. If you start to gain a bit of weight, that is okay! It just means your metabolism is working again!

Proteins (palm of hand)	Fats (tablespoon)	Carbohydrates (fist)	Vegetables (fist)
4 oz chicken breast	2 tbsp nut butter	3/4 cup sweet potato	Broccoli
4 oz turkey breast	1 tbsp coconut oil	1/2 cup beans/ legumes	Cauliflower
4 oz fish	1 tbsp olive oil	1/2 cup brown rice	Peppers
1 can tuna	1/2 avocado	1 slice bread	Squash
1/2 cup Greek yogurt	1 tbsp seeds	1/2 cup oats	Spinach
1/2 cup cottage cheese	12 almonds	1/2 cup pasta	Bok choy
1 cup egg whites	1 tbsp butter	1/2 cup quinoa	Kale
4 oz shellfish	1 tbsp coffee cream	3/4 berries	Green beans

Ensuring you get enough energy through food is the first and most crucial step to ensuring your metabolism functions properly, which can aid in weight loss. Other factors that affect our BMR include the amount of water we drink, the duration and quality of our sleep, and our thyroid function.

Interestingly, drinking enough water can temporarily boost your metabolic rate. You may have heard that drinking water is important for weight loss. This is true because your body needs to heat the water you drink, and this process burns energy, possibly up to 400 calories! One study found that drinking 500 mL of water increased metabolism by 30%, and this effect lasted for about 30–40 minutes [4].

Sleep also plays a critical role. Compared to those who sleep less than seven hours per night, people who sleep more than 7 hours lose more weight, even if they eat the same things and exercise the same amount [5]. This is because a lack of sleep slows down our metabolism [6]. Poor sleep can also increase food cravings. Have you ever felt like you want to snack more when you are really tired? This is because a lack of sleep disrupts our appetite control centers in our brain [7]. There's a dedicated chapter on improving sleep, which may be worth exploring if this is a challenge for you.

Another piece of the puzzle for BMR is thyroid health, and anyone on a weight loss journey will require thorough thyroid testing to ensure it is functioning correctly. Refer to Chapter 5 on thyroid dysfunction for detailed guidance and suggested blood work.

CLINICAL PEARL

Here's a small checklist to ensure your BMR is working correctly:

- Calculate your BMR at www.calculator.net;
- Make sure you're consuming enough calories and eating the foods listed in the provided table;
- Lift weights two to three days per week;
- Drink at least 2 L of water daily;
- Get at least seven hours of sleep each night; and
- Have your thyroid checked.

Step 2: Mentally Commit

This step might be the most crucial of all. You may need to break free from food addictions and become highly aware of the emotional triggers that prompt you to reach for the cupboard. You might also need to relearn to be curious about the flavors and textures of foods, and to consistently remind yourself of the dangers of processed foods.

You might need to break free from the temptation of immediate pleasure from foods and intellectually understand how certain habits have become deeply ingrained within you. All of this calls for strong self-awareness, compassion, and mindfulness.

In the book "If the Buddha Came to Dinner," when you feel the urge to eat as an emotional response, Schaltz advises you to ask yourself, "Who am I feeding?" Are you feeding anger, sadness, or stress? Or are you nourishing your true self, your "honored guest"? This reflection helps increase awareness of emotional eating patterns that often hinder weight loss goals.

Mindful eating involves paying full attention to your food while you eat. This means noticing the colors, aromas, and textures of food, eating slowly, and taking pauses between bites. It takes approximately 15–20 minutes for the brain to realize when we are full after we start eating. Therefore, it is recommended to spread out meals over at least 15 minutes to allow your body to signal when it is full. Mindful eating encourages you to slow down and savor your food.

Tasting a Strawberry for the First Time

You're sitting in the kitchen, craving a snack. You head to the fridge and recall the delicious, ripe strawberries you bought. You grab a few from the container and sit down to enjoy them.

First, examine the strawberries. Are the green tops still attached? Are they uniformly red, or do they have some yellow spots? You notice their varying sizes and shapes.

Next, select one and hold it in your palm. Is it wet or rough? Did it roll around? Examine it as if you've never seen a strawberry in your entire life.

Hold the strawberry close to your nose and breathe in its aroma. Does it smell delightfully ripe, or does it need more time? Does it make your mouth water?

Now is the time to taste it. Touch it to your lips. Feel the seeds. Maybe you hold the strawberry in your mouth before biting down. Is it juicy? Sour? Sweet? Chew slowly until it is in small pieces, then swallow.

To help you mentally commit to your weight loss goals, knowing your "why" and connecting to deeper drives can boost lasting motivation. Instead of focusing on numbers on a scale, think about why you want to lose weight—whether to have more energy, feel stronger after cancer, improve sleep, or manage health conditions. Writing these reasons down and revisiting them often helps maintain motivation.

Start small and set realistic goals—you don't need to make sweeping changes all at once. Perhaps your first goal is to walk for 15 minutes three times a week or to incorporate one extra serving of vegetables into your daily meals. As you achieve these smaller wins, it builds momentum and confidence. Celebrate each success, no matter how small! There will be days when you don't stick perfectly to your plan, and that's okay. It's part of the process. Remember, it's about the overall trend of progress, not daily perfection.

What you say to yourself is important, so make sure to foster positive self-talk. Be kind and compassionate to yourself. Negative self-talk undermines progress. Instead, concentrate on your strengths and the positive changes you are making. Affirmations like "I am making healthy choices for myself" or "I am getting stronger every day" can be powerful.

Visualization is also a powerful tool. Take a moment to envision yourself achieving your goals and how that will feel. Visualize having more energy, feeling stronger, and enjoying the activities you love. The more vividly you can see yourself succeeding, the more likely you are to stay the course.

This journey isn't always easy. Be patient and understanding with yourself. If you have a setback, acknowledge it without judgment and gently redirect your focus. Remember that this is not a sprint. It's a lifelong journey of learning and growth.

Step 3: Choose an Eating Pattern and Stick with It

Here's a surprising truth: there doesn't seem to be a magic way of eating that guarantees weight loss. A substantial amount of research has been conducted to determine the most effective eating patterns. What research has shown is that most eating patterns can help you lose weight, as long as you stick with them and don't become impatient.

Large-scale studies comparing low-carb, low-fat, and high-protein diets have all shown that they can be effective. Mediterranean, ketogenic, and intermittent fasting patterns have all produced favorable outcomes for weight loss. As mentioned elsewhere in this book, the goal is to nourish the body, and any kind of restrictive diet, such as low-calorie diets, is not recommended here, as they carry a high risk of weight regain and are generally not enjoyable.

Intermittent Fasting

Nearly all studies on intermittent fasting (IF) have produced positive weight loss results, ranging from 2.5 to 10% body weight loss [8]. Popular IF protocols include the 5:2 method (where you eat normally for five days and restrict calories for two days) and alternate-day fasting (where you eat normally one day, then fast the next day).

A recent research review found that individuals who regularly use intermittent fasting may lose up to 10 pounds of body weight [9]. Beyond weight loss, fat mass is reduced, blood sugar levels are lowered, cholesterol levels are reduced, waist circumference decreases, and measures of inflammation improve [10].

One of the benefits of IF is that it doesn't limit the types of food you can eat. While a whole-foods approach is always ideal, rich in lean protein, fiber, healthy fats, and plant-based foods, you don't need to count every calorie or cut out entire food groups.

Low-fat vs. Low-carb vs. Mediterranean Diet

Each eating pattern takes a slightly different approach. The food pyramids below can help you visualize the comparisons between different nutritional styles.

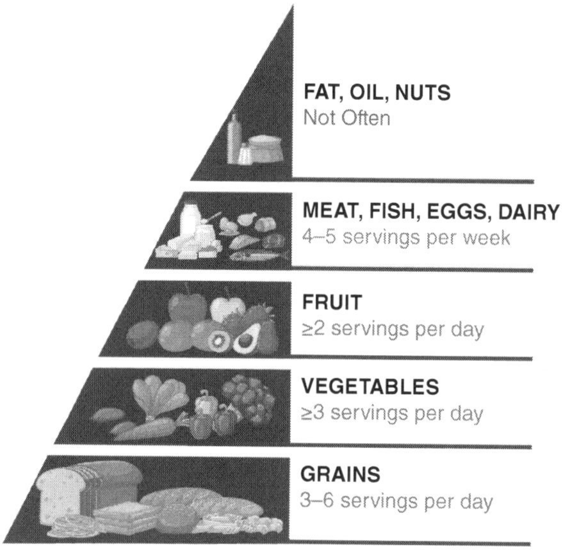

LOW FAT DIET

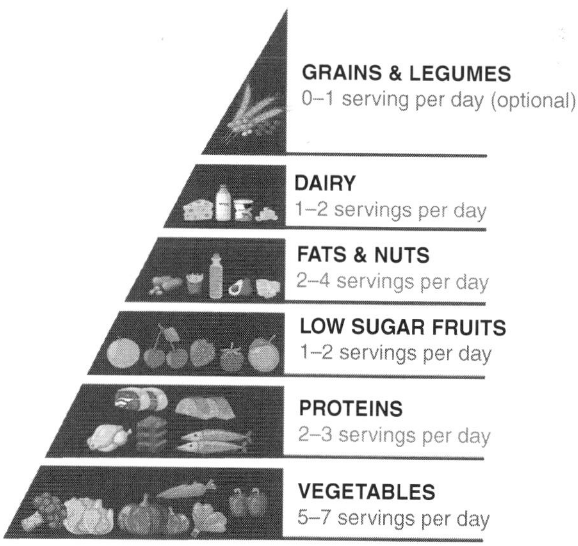

LOW CARBOHYDRATE DIET

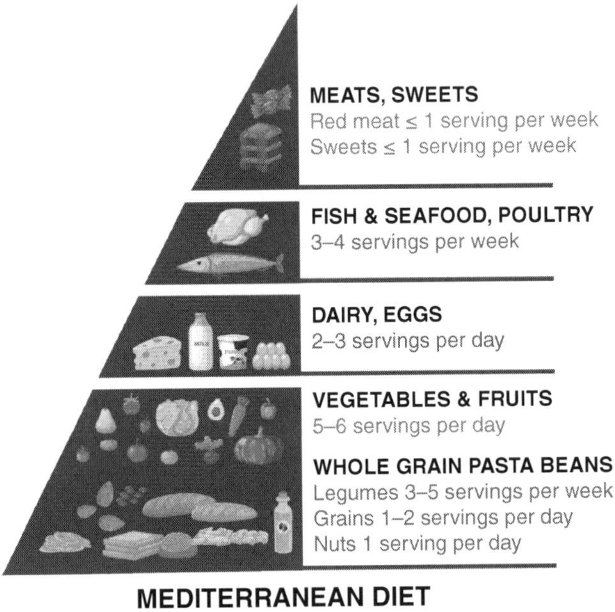

An interesting study compared the effectiveness of various eating patterns for weight loss [11]. What was notable is that participants were allowed to choose their preferred way of eating. Because preferences were considered, adherence remained high at the two-year follow-up, with 85% of participants following the guidelines.

Weight loss occurred in all three groups, with the most significant results seen in the low-carb and Mediterranean diet groups. The low-fat group lost an average of 6–15 pounds. The Mediterranean diet group lost 10–22 pounds. The low-carb group achieved a loss of 10–26 pounds.

Each group also experienced reductions in waist circumference, blood pressure, and cholesterol levels. However, only the low-carb and Mediterranean groups saw a decrease in inflammation.

If you eat a high amount of carbohydrates by way of bread, grains, and pasta, a low-carb diet will likely be very successful for you. Otherwise, the Mediterranean diet is generally the best all-around choice, thanks to its anti-inflammatory benefits. Just make sure not to go over your daily calorie limit, as determined by your BMR calculation. Chapter 4 further explains serving sizes to ensure you stay within your limits.

Mediterranean Diet vs. Healthy Ketogenic Diet

These eating patterns are similar in that they are healthy fat-forward and allow high lean protein, but they differ in carbohydrate content. A study compared these two methods of eating and their impact on weight loss [12]. The food pyramids below will allow you to visualize the comparisons more easily.

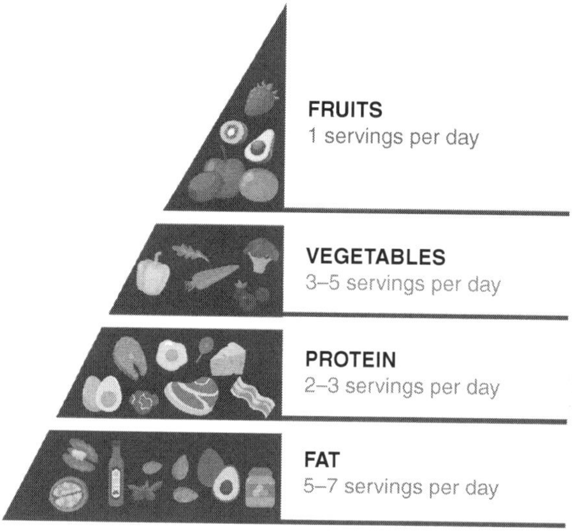

KETO DIET

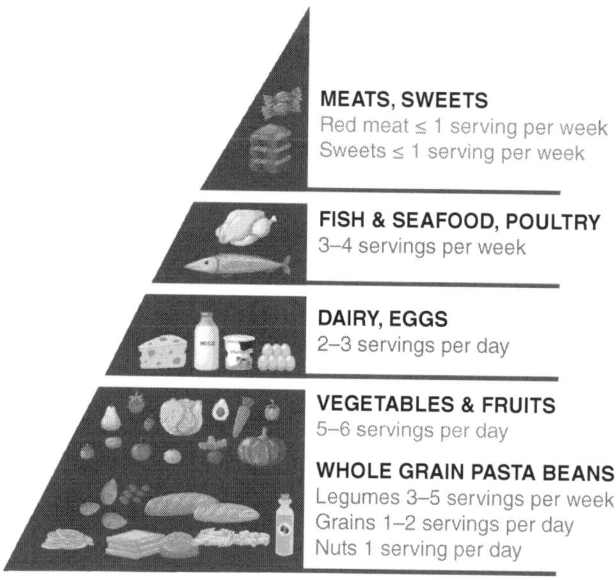

MEDITERRANEAN DIET

After three months, the researchers found that both eating patterns led to significant weight loss, but waist circumference decreased more in the Mediterranean diet group. However, the ketogenic diet resulted in faster weight loss.

As discussed in Chapter 4, a ketogenic diet is likely low in fruits and vegetables, which is the main reason this author does not recommend the long-term use of the ketogenic diet for weight loss. If you need to lose weight quickly, this approach can be effective; however, for lasting success and sustainability, the Mediterranean diet may be a better choice.

Success Story

Mark was a 30-year-old man who was a survivor of childhood cancer. He had gained a significant amount of weight during his 20s, which he attributed to poor lifestyle choices. He came to see me for joint pain, indigestion, headaches, depression, and fatigue. His main goal was weight loss, and I challenged him to lose 8 pounds per month over six months, and all of his complaints would improve.

He was highly motivated, and to help him achieve quick results, I recommended the healthy ketogenic diet outlined above. He mostly ate fish, nuts and seeds, eggs, chicken, and vegetables for two months. We concentrated on nutrition, as his knee and lower back pain limited his physical activity during this period. He started acupuncture for pain management, and after one month, he was able to begin swimming, an activity he found relaxing and that reduced his stress.

After two months on the ketogenic diet, he lost 22 pounds. However, he grew tired of his meal choices and switched to a more Mediterranean diet, incorporating more fruits and yogurt. After a total of six months, he had lost 41 pounds. He no longer complained of indigestion, his joint pain was 90% better, he no longer experienced headaches, and he felt more confident and happy. He was pleased to report that his energy had skyrocketed.

Step 4: Determine Your Daily Activity Routine

When it comes to weight loss, it is generally believed that your nutritional choices are more important for shedding pounds, while physical activity helps to maintain the loss. However, it is wise to include physical activity throughout the weight loss journey. Lifting weights helps to build muscle, which boosts your BMR. Losing weight without building muscle may leave you feeling weak rather than energized.

Physical activity guidelines vary, but at a minimum, it is recommended to engage in 150 minutes of exercise per week. For more substantial weight loss,

300 minutes of exercise per week is optimal. That equates to 60 minutes a day, five days a week! This weight loss will directly lead to increased energy. Vigorous physical activity will also boost your mood and help you sleep better.

If vigorous workouts feel out of reach right now, consider incorporating light to moderate-intensity activities, such as brisk walking, water aerobics, or dancing. The table below can guide you on what is considered vigorous or moderate intensity. As discussed in Chapter 8, it seems not to matter what kind of physical activity you take part in—choose something you enjoy, and do it most days of the week.

Moderate level activities	
Dancing	Jumping on a mini trampoline
Badminton	Kayaking
Baseball	Raking leaves
Shooting hoops	Shoveling snow
Leisurely biking	Downhill skiing
Walking	Tai chi
Gardening	Tennis
Ice skating	Volleyball
Vigorous level activities	
Vigorous basketball game	Rollerblading
Biking 20 km/hour	Soccer
Touch football	Swimming
Ultimate frisbee	Speed walking
Hockey	Climbing stairs
Jogging or running	Water polo
Racquetball	Cross-country skiing
Hiking	Jumping rope

Tracking Your Progress and Staying on Track

Assess Your Body Composition

Tracking your progress can boost motivation and help you refine your approach. If you plan to monitor your progress solely with a traditional weight scale, check your weight only once per month.

Assessing your body fat percentage and muscle mass is ideal. While some devices might be harder to access, obtaining a requisition for a DEXA scan or visiting a clinic with a body impedance analysis (BIA) scale can effectively measure your muscle and fat mass. General guidelines are available to help you determine healthy ranges based on your gender and age. Women should aim for a body fat percentage between 18 and 28%, whereas men should aim for 10–20%.

The body mass index (BMI) is a calculation based on your sex, height, and weight, and the score generally indicates whether you are in the recommended healthy range. However, this can sometimes be inaccurate for individuals with a high level of muscle mass, as muscle weighs more than fat. Typically, a score between 18.5 and 25 indicates a healthy range.

Waist circumference is a simple measurement that can be taken at home. Using a soft tape measure, wrap it around your torso at the level of your belly button. Men should aim for a waist measurement of under 102 cm, and women should aim for a measurement of under 88 cm. You can also take measurements of your upper arms or upper thighs to observe changes there.

Track Evidence of Success Beyond the Number on the Scale

Revisit your list of reasons why you wanted to lose weight in the first place. Was it to have more energy to play with your kids? Was it to experience less knee pain? Was it to feel more confident in your clothes? Was it to help manage high blood pressure or blood sugar?

Check this list daily! Record the changes and improvements you notice, including your feelings and emotions. By writing down tangible changes, you'll start to focus on the real ways your quality of life is improving, rather than just the number on the scale.

Here are some examples of ways to track evidence of success:

- Fasting blood sugar reading week 1 __, fasting blood sugar reading week 3 __;
- Hours slept per night in week 1 __, hours slept per night in week 3 __;
- Knee pain week 1 __, knee pain week 3 __;
- How tired did I feel after playing tag with kids in week 1 __, and how tired did I feel in week 3 __?
- Comfort of favorite jeans week 1 __, comfort of favorite jeans week 3 __.

Whatever your why, find meaningful ways to track your progress, aiming to observe these changes over at least six months. Celebrate minor improvements, as each one contributes to significant long-term results.

Mindset for Lasting Change

If you find your weight loss efforts slow or minimal, remember what it was like saving for your retirement or a trip. Each small deposit might feel insignificant at the time, but over the long haul, those efforts add up to something powerful. Weight loss works the same way; your efforts are laying the foundation for lasting health. Do not get discouraged with minimal or slow results.

Many of us hold beliefs like "I'll never lose weight" or "I'm just destined to be heavy." Reframe these thoughts into empowering affirmations, such as "I'm strong because I make healthy choices" or "My body deserves the utmost nourishment and respect." These mindset shifts are subtle but powerful. They foster resilience and help keep you grounded when old patterns reappear.

Earlier in this chapter, we discussed the power of visualization. Picture yourself happily moving around the kitchen, chopping vegetables and grilling some delicious chicken. Imagine the wonderful smells and how pleased you are to sit down and slowly enjoy the meal you've made. These kinds of visualizations are useful and strong to keep in your mind, so that you can use them to cancel out thoughts about wanting foods that no longer serve you.

Visualization and unconditional positive self-talk are essential for cultivating a healthier relationship with food and achieving lasting weight loss, fostering a sense of empowerment. Remember, the key is to view your weight loss journey not as a temporary effort or a quick fix, but as a meaningful lifestyle shift, making the journey feel less like a battle and more like a natural progression toward your best self.

Conclusion

It's no surprise that navigating weight loss can feel incredibly confusing. The sheer volume of conflicting advice can leave anyone unsure where to begin. But truly effective weight loss isn't about deprivation. It's about feeding your body and mind.

The first step is to prioritize foods that genuinely energize you and that you truly enjoy. Secondly, you must eliminate all processed foods and sugary drinks entirely. These will sabotage both your waistline and your energy. And most importantly, consistency is your greatest ally.

Achieving a healthier weight can dramatically boost your energy levels by easing the physical strain on your entire body. If you're uncertain about how to eat for effective weight loss, start by embracing any of the nourishing eating patterns outlined in the food pyramids presented earlier in this book. These aren't fleeting fad diets—they are sustainable, whole-food approaches designed to support you. As you begin, pay close attention to the shifts in your energy, improvements in your sleep and mood, and feel the powerful changes in your physical well-being.

References

1 Bleich S, Cutler D, Murray C, et al. Why is the developed world obese? Annu Rev Public Health, 2008; 29:273–295.
2 Poti JM, Braga B, Qin B. Ultra-processed food intake and obesity: what really matters for health—processing or nutrient content?. Curr Obes Rep, 2017; 6:420–431.
3 Lane M, Gamage E, Du S, et al. Ultra-processed food exposure and adverse health outcomes: umbrella review of epidemiological meta-analyses. BMJ, 2024; 384:e077310.
4 Boschmann M, Steiniger J, Hille U, et al. Water-induced thermogenesis. J Clin Endocr Metab, 2003; 88(12):6015–6019.
5 Thomson CA, Morrow KI, Flatt SW, et al. Relationship between sleep quality and quantity and weight loss in women participating in a weight-loss intervention trial. Obesity, 2012; 20:1419–1425.
6 Nedeltcheva AV, Kilkus JM, Imperial J, et al. Insuffiicient sleep undermines dietary efforts to reduce adiposity. Ann Intern Med, 2010; 153:435–411.
7 Taheri S, Lin L, Austin D, et al. Short sleep duration is associated with reduce leptin, elevated ghrelin, and increased body mass index. PLoS Med, 2004; 1:e62.
8 Byrne NMM, Sainsbury A, King NAA, et al. Intermittent energy restriction improves weight loss efficiency in obese men: the MATADOR study. Int J Obes (Lond), 2018; 42(2):129-138.
9 Almabruk BA, Alharbi SH, Alsaqer FS, et al. The role of intermittent fasting on metabolic syndrome: a systematic review and meta-analysis. Cureus, 2024; 16(10):e71623.
10 Stockman MC, Thomas D, Burke J, et al. Intermittent fasting: is the wait worth the weight?. Curr Obes Rep, 2019; 7(2):172–185.
11 Shai I, Schwarzfuchs D, Henkin Y, et al. Weight loss with a low-carbohydrate, Mediterranean, or low-fat diet. N Engl J Med, 2008; 359:229–241.
12 Di Rosa C, Lattanzi G, Spiezia C, et al. Mediterranean diet versus very low-calorie ketogenic diet: effects of reaching 5% body weight loss on body composition in subject with overweight and with obesity—a cohort study. Int J Environ Res Public Health, 2022; 19(20):13040.

10

Healthy Weight Gain for Nourishing Your Comeback

It's not until you get tired that you see how strong you really are

—Shaun T

This chapter is for you if:

- You have experienced unintentional weight loss due to your illness, especially muscle loss, and are struggling with weakness and fatigue.
- You have lost weight due to side effects of cancer treatments, such as nausea, loss of appetite, constipation, diarrhea, or changes in taste.

Before starting cancer treatment, people often hear from doctors and nurses, "don't lose weight." This may seem confusing, as Chapter 9 emphasized the importance of weight loss. The key difference is the type of weight being lost. In Chapter 9, we focused on losing fat specifically, as well as on maintaining or gaining muscle mass to support weight loss if you are overweight or obese.

The type of weight loss we're discussing here can be dangerous, mainly involving the loss of muscle tissue. This condition is called cancer cachexia and is characterized by a progressive, often difficult-to-treat weight loss of more than 5% of body weight over six months. The significance of this issue is highlighted by its statistics—about 50–80% of people with cancer will experience cachexia [1]. It leads to a poor quality of life and increases the risk of death.

Cancer cachexia is vitally important to address because it causes severe fatigue, which limits physical activity and contributes to muscle weakness. Weight loss can cause distressing mental fatigue as the physical changes that can occur take a toll on patients' emotions. Low muscle mass decreases quality of life and is linked with depression, which worsens fatigue [2]. Research indicates that gaining weight, in this context, is associated with improved survival [3].

Beyond Cancer Fatigue: A Path to Reclaiming Energy, First Edition. Jessa Landmann, ND.

Weight loss does not occur solely from eating less food. It involves a chronic inflammatory state caused by cancer itself and its treatments. This inflammation can lead to mitochondrial dysfunction in the muscles, reducing the energy produced by muscle tissue. Additionally, inflammation increases the risk of developing insulin resistance and diabetes, which means that insufficient fuel enters the body's cells.

Hormonal imbalances, particularly elevated cortisol levels, also play a role. When inflammation is high, cortisol, our stress hormone, is released. Cortisol contributes to poor blood sugar control and also breaks down muscle [4].

Cancer also doesn't use energy very efficiently. Think of cancer as a "hungry tumor," and because it grows quickly and diverts energy away from the rest of the body, it contributes to fatigue and muscle wasting.

All of this together—the inflammation, the disrupted hormones, and the increased energy requirement—results in muscle loss, weakness, and profound fatigue. These physical changes and potential loss of independence may lead to psychological distress, depression, and anxiety, which makes energy levels even lower.

Other reasons for weight loss in those with cancer are a result of side effects from cancer treatments, such as nausea, constipation, diarrhea, lack of appetite, and taste changes. Stomach pain and mouth sores may also be present, and all these together create the perfect environment for weight loss to occur, placing individuals at long-term risk of nutritional deficiencies and low energy.

That is why, to combat cachexia, it's not just about eating more food. Since the causes of cachexia are multifaceted, treatment must be too. Let's explore some complementary therapies you can start considering today.

Complementary Therapies for Cachexia

Address Insulin Resistance

One of the first steps in addressing unexpected or uncontrollable weight loss is to check for insulin resistance. When the body becomes resistant to insulin, it has a harder time using sugar and protein from food for energy and muscle repair. As a result, even if a person is eating enough, their body may continue to break down muscle and lose strength. By identifying and addressing insulin resistance early, it may be possible to help the body use nutrients more efficiently, support muscle maintenance, and slow further weight loss. Suggested blood work and treatments are found in Chapter 8. Several supplements are highly effective at reducing insulin resistance, and my primary recommendation is berberine [5].

CLINICAL PEARL

Berberine at a dose of 500 mg three times daily may help with insulin resistance. However, if severe fatigue, dizziness, or increased nausea occurs, reduce the dose to 500 mg twice daily.

Fish Oil (EPA)

EPA is an omega-3 fatty acid found in fish oil that has potent anti-inflammatory effects. As reducing inflammation is one of the primary objectives for reversing cachexia, this is an important supplement to incorporate.

A large clinical trial enrolled 200 patients with stage II–IV pancreatic cancer who were suffering from cachexia [6]. Half of the participants received high-dose EPA fish oil supplements, while the other half did not. After the completion of the 12-week trial, analysis revealed that individuals who took fish oil experienced a significant increase in body weight and an increase in muscle mass. These results have been replicated in other small trials [7].

CLINICAL PEARL

A high EPA-containing fish oil supplement is the key. Doses of EPA alone should be at least 2.2 g. It is essential to examine the label and verify the EPA dose specifically, not just the total fish oil content.

L-Carnitine

L-Carnitine is an amino acid that plays a vital role in energy production within the mitochondria. Muscle tissue is usually rich in carnitine, but people suffering from cancer cachexia have low levels [8]. One trial of individuals experiencing weight loss who received a daily supplement of L-carnitine found that after 12 weeks, body weight significantly increased [9].

CLINICAL PEARL

Since weight and muscle gain take time, remember to stay consistent for several months. A dose of 4 g of L-carnitine is recommended, and this is one of the most reliable supplements that can assist.

Success Story

Andre was diagnosed with tongue cancer and had lost a significant amount of weight due to reduced food intake caused by mouth pain. He had completed radiation therapy and was making good progress with rehab. However, his energy levels were very low, and he struggled to get through the day at work.

He was struggling with dry mouth and difficulty swallowing and couldn't consume enough food to regain the weight he lost. He told me he did not find it difficult to swallow pills with enough water. I recommended 4 g of L-carnitine and 2 g of fish oil daily. After two months, he was able to gain 6 pounds of muscle without changing his diet.

β-Hydroxy β-Methylbutyrate (HMB)

This is another oral supplement that has great potential to support weight gain and muscle development. HMB simultaneously activates pathways in the body that promote muscle growth, as well as those that prevent the breakdown of existing muscle [10]. In individuals with cancer, HMB helps increase muscle mass, resulting in a higher body weight and an improved quality of life [11].

CLINICAL PEARL

A daily dose of 3 g of HMB, taken consistently for at least three months, is a valuable addition to a comprehensive cachexia recovery plan.

Dietary Protein Intake

Consuming sufficient protein is essential to preserving and rebuilding muscle mass. Most guidelines recommend that patients with cancer cachexia aim for 1.0–1.5 g of protein per kilogram body weight; however, an intake exceeding 1.5 g per kilogram is recommended [12].

Animal proteins, such as meat, poultry, fish, eggs, and dairy, are among the richest sources of protein. However, consuming such a high volume of meat and animal products may be difficult for many patients, especially those with poor appetite and nausea. In these cases, protein powder smoothies can serve as a great alternative to help meet protein goals.

Whey protein is the preferred supplement for supporting muscle growth and aids in weight regain in people recovering from cancer treatment [13]. Whey is rich in the amino acid leucine, which is one of three branched-chain amino acids (BCAAs) that act as a "trigger" for anabolic, or muscle-building, potential [14].

One study provided participants with 40 g of whey protein, 4.16 g of leucine, and fish oil and found statistically significant increases in muscle mass [15]. This highlights the potential benefit of using multiple nutritional therapies in combination, rather than relying on a single strategy.

CLINICAL PEARL

Find a high-quality whey protein powder and add 40 g per day to your smoothie of choice.

Physical Activity

For muscles to grow, they must be used. It can seem like an enormous challenge for someone dealing with muscle weakness and fatigue to find the motivation to exercise. Something as simple as standing up and sitting down from a chair 10 times, several times a day, can help. Wall push-ups are another gentle way to engage your muscles.

Researchers have reported that training just a few muscles can help gain muscle and body weight and combat dangerous weight loss [16]. Just a few exercises, such as knee extensions and bicep and tricep curls, for three months are enough to help build muscle mass, especially if energy levels are low [17].

It is very important not to do anything unsafe, like climbing stairs, where balance or falling could cause someone to seriously hurt themselves. It is best to ask a qualified trainer or other health professional for advice. Additionally, later in this book, you will find a dedicated chapter on muscle building with more detailed guidance.

Hydration

Theoretically, proper hydration supports muscle recovery and boosts energy levels. Dehydration can worsen muscle fatigue by reducing blood flow and oxygen delivery to muscle tissue. Some community studies have found that older adults with low water intake tend to have lower muscle mass than those with adequate hydration [18]. A goal is to drink at least 2 L of water daily. More may be necessary in hot weather or if you are physically active. Make hydration a part of your daily health routine.

Complementary Therapies for Other Side Effects That Can Contribute to Weight Loss

Nausea

Ginger

Ginger should be one of the first remedies to try if nausea interferes with your ability to eat properly. Interestingly, ginger acts similarly to prescription nausea medication. It is safe, has minimal side effects, and is highly effective for nausea [19].

Capsules are far superior, as they provide a precise dose that can't be matched by ginger teas, ginger chews, or grating ginger into food.

CLINICAL PEARL

Look for a capsule with a dose ranging from 300 to 500 mg, and take them one to five times per day, or as needed.

Acupuncture

At a pharmacy, ask about a product called a Sea Band. These bracelets apply pressure to a specific acupuncture point on the inner forearm, effectively alleviating nausea. Alternatively, if you can see an acupuncturist, a comprehensive treatment plan can also be beneficial.

CLINICAL PEARL

My protocol for treating nausea with acupuncture is as follows: PC6, ST25, CV12, CV20, SP15, ST36, GB21.

Loss of Appetite

Bitters

It is never advisable to force yourself to eat when your appetite is low. This can create negative feelings toward food and lead to further eating issues. Bitter herbs have been used for centuries in traditional medicine to stimulate appetite and digestion. The idea behind why bitters work is that the bitter receptors on the tongue increase saliva production and send signals to other digestive organs that food is on its way. Bitters boost digestive secretions and enhance blood flow to organs, which also helps stimulate appetite [20].

CLINICAL PEARL

Classic bitters that are used to stimulate the appetite include black coffee, gentian, and wormwood. Just 2 ml about 15 minutes before a meal can help.

THC

THC is an extract from the cannabis plant and has shown effectiveness in increasing appetite across a variety of clinical settings. Most studies have found positive results for helping to increase body weight, and it is safe, even in the elderly [21].

CLINICAL PEARL

Start with a dose of 2.5 mg THC, and increase to 5 mg if the psychoactive effects do not deter you.

Loss of Taste

Zinc

Changes in taste after cancer treatment can be very distressing and are often underestimated. When food no longer tastes right, meals can feel like a chore instead of a comfort, and favorite dishes may suddenly seem unappealing. Taste is one of the great pleasures of life and an important part of recovery—it not only makes eating enjoyable but also stimulates appetite and supports good nutrition. A simple zinc swish and swallow can be quite effective, often with lasting results [22].

CLINICAL PEARL

Buy an affordable zinc tablet, around 5 mg, at a pharmacy. Crush the tablet, mix it with water, swish for 30 seconds, then swallow. Repeat this a few times daily until the taste returns.

Constipation

Chronic constipation can decrease appetite because when the colon is backed up, it can cause people to feel full and nauseous, which reduces the desire to eat. Constipation is very common after cancer treatment, but several things can help.

Senna

Senna is a plant native to parts of Africa and Asia, and it is gentle, effective, and non-habit-forming for people dealing with constipation. It can be taken in capsule or tea form.

> **CLINICAL PEARL**
>
> Find an over-the-counter senna product with a dosage of 8.6 mg per tablet. These are best taken at night so they can work while you sleep. Smooth Move tea is a popular brand that allows you to enjoy senna as a soothing hot beverage.

Magnesium

Two forms of magnesium can help draw water into the bowel and facilitate easier bowel movements: magnesium oxide and magnesium citrate. Both are effective, and dosages vary between individuals. It is best to start with a low dose and gradually increase to avoid cramping or loose stools, then adjust until you find what works best for you.

> **CLINICAL PEARL**
>
> Begin with a dose of 400 mg and gradually increase up to 1.5 g. It is advisable to take magnesium at night so it can work through your system while you sleep.

Information for Health Care Professionals

Cachexia can be a distressing symptom and a palliative challenge for healthcare providers. It is advised to perform a blood test for albumin and C-reactive protein (CRP), as these markers can be used to calculate the Glasgow Prognostic Score (GPS) for classifying cachexia. This score can be calculated using online tools and has been shown to offer clinically meaningful assessments for different stages of cachexia: no cachexia, undernourished, pre-cachexia, and refractory cachexia [23].

These blood tests can be useful, especially when dealing with sarcopenia and obesity. Due to the high prevalence of overweight and obesity, it can be difficult to visually detect significant weight loss, particularly muscle loss, in individuals with excess adipose tissue. Using a DEXA machine or BIA scale will also help in identifying muscle loss in this group.

Other useful tests include fasting insulin and fasting glucose to detect insulin resistance, as well as morning cortisol levels. Both of these factors contribute to cachexia and fatigue and can be targeted using the strategies outlined throughout this book.

References

1 Fearon K, Strasser F, Anker SD, et al. Definition and classification of cancer cachexia: an international consensus. Lancet Oncol, 2011; 12(5):489–495.

2 Nipp RD, Fuchs G, El-Jawahri A, et al. Sarcopenia is associated with quality of life and depression in patients with advanced cancer. Oncologist, 2018; 23:97–104.

3 Roeland EJ, Fintelmann FJ, Hilton F, et al. The relationship between weight gain during chemotherapy and outcomes in patients with advanced non-small cell lung cancer. J Each Sarc Must, 2024; 15(3):1030–1040.

4 Shimizu N, Yoshikawa N, Ito N, et al. Crosstalk between glucocorticoid receptor and nutritional sensor mTOR in skeletal muscle. Cell Metab, 2011; 13:170–182.

5 Bellavite P, Fazio S. Affuso F. A descriptive review of the action mechanisms of berberine, quercetin and silymarin on insulin resistance/hyperinsulinemia and cardiovascular prevention. Molecules, 2023; 28:491.

6 Fearon KCH, von Meyenfeldt MF, Moses, AGW, et al. Effect of a protein and energy dense N-3 fatty acid enriched oral supplement on loss of weight and lean tissue in cancer cachexia: a randomized- double blind trial. Gut, 2003; 52:1479–1486.

7 Akita H, Takahashi H, Asukai K, et al. The utility of nutritional supportive care with an EPA enriched nutrition agent during pre-op chemoradiotherapy for pancreatic cancer: prospective randomized control study. Clin Nutr ESPEN, 2019; 33:148–153.

8 Vinci E, Rampello E, Zanoli L, et al. Serum carnitine levels in patients with tumoral cachexia. Eur J Intern Med, 2005; 16:419–423.

9 Kraft M, Kraft K, Gartner S, et al. Carnitine supplementation in advanced pancreatic cancer (CARPAN) – a randomized multi centre trial. Nutr J, 2012; 11:52.

10 Wilkinson DJ, Hossain T, Hill DS, et al. Effects of leucine and its metabolite β-hydroxy-β-methylbutyrate on human skeletal muscle protein metabolism. J Physiol, 2013; 591:2911–2923.

11 Prado CM, Orsso CE, Pereira SL, et al. Effects of B-hydroxy B-methylbutyrate (HMB) supplementation on muscle mass, function, and other outcomes in patients with cancer: a systematic review. J Cach Sarc Musc, 2022; 13(3):1623–1641.

12 Op den Kamp CM, Langen RC, Haegens A, et al. Muscle atrophy in cachexia: can dietary protein tip the balance. Curr Opin Clin Nutr Metab Care, 2009; 12:611–616.
13 Sahni S, Mangano KM, Hannan MT, et al. Higher protein intake is associated with higher lean mass and quadriceps muscle strength in adult men and women. J Nutr, 2015; 145(7):1569–1575.
14 Barone M, Baccaro P, Molfino A. An overview of sarcopenia: focusing on nutritional treatment approaches. Nutrients, 2025; 17(7):1237.
15 Deutz NE, Safar A, Schutzler S, et al. Muscle protein synthesis in cancer patients can be stimulated with a specially formulated medical food. Clin Nutr, 2011; 30(6):759–768.
16 Mavropalias G, Sim M, Taaffe DR, et al. Exercise medicine for cancer cachexia: targeted exercise to counteract mechanisms and treatment side effects. J Cancer Res Clin Oncol, 2022; 148:1389–1406.
17 Kamel FH, Basha MA, Alsharidah AS, et al. Resistance training impact on mobility, muscle strength and lean mass in pancreatic cancer cachexia: a randomized controlled trial. Clin Rehabil, 2020; 34(11):1391–1399.
18 Yoo JI, Choi H, Song SY, et al. Relationship between water intake and skeletal muscle mass in elderly Koreans: a nationwide population-based study. Nutrition, 2018; 53:38–42.
19 Lin CY, Huang SH, Tam KW, et al. Efficacy and safety of ginger on chemotherapy-induced nausea and vomiting: a systematic review and meta-analysis of randomized controlled trials. Cancer Nurs, 2024; 48(6):455–466.
20 McMullen MK, Whitehouse JM, Towell A. Bitters: time for a new paradigm. Evid Based Complement Alternat Med, 2015; 2015:670504.
21 Ceolin C, De Rui M, Ravelli A, et al. The potential of cannabinoids in managing cancer-related anorexia in older adults: a systematic review of the literature. J Nutr Health Aging, 2024; 28(8):100299.
22 Spencer AS, da Silva Dias D, Capelas ML, et al. Managing severe dysgeusia and dysosmia in lung cancer patients: a systematic scoping review. Front Oncol, 2021; 11:774081.
23 Burgassi F, Paillaud E, Poisson J, et al. Prognostic value of prospective longitudinal CRP to albumin ratio among older outpatients with cancer. Cancers (Basel), 2021; 13(22):5782.

Part IV

Mental and Emotional Causes of Cancer-related Fatigue

11

Lifting the Cloud of Depression

There is no health without mental health

—David Satcher, former US Surgeon General

A sad soul is as lethal as a germ

—John Steinbeck

This chapter is for you if:

- You feel sad or emotionally low as a result of your cancer experience and everything you've been through.
- You notice depression affecting other areas of your life, and you want to stop the negative cycle.
- You are taking antidepressant medication and want to explore whether complementary therapies can help.

Depression casts a long shadow, not only as a widespread global concern but particularly for those navigating the complex journey of cancer. For individuals undergoing treatment or in survivorship, the risk of experiencing depression soars—nearly four times higher than the general population. This critical reality underscores a vital truth: proactive and consistent screening for depression is essential, not just at diagnosis, but continuously through treatment and into recovery.

Addressing depression is a pivotal step, as its presence can profoundly diminish quality of life, intensifying fatigue, disrupting healthy eating and exercise routines, and stealing restorative sleep. By acknowledging and addressing these interconnected challenges, we open a powerful pathway to reignite energy and foster emotional well-being for cancer survivors.

Beyond Cancer Fatigue: A Path to Reclaiming Energy, First Edition. Jessa Landmann, ND.

Depression is a common and complex challenge that many face after a cancer diagnosis. Biologically, it can stem from inflammation caused by chemotherapy or changes in sex hormone levels. Emotionally, survivors often mourn their "old life," feeling isolated and misunderstood. They may also grapple with trauma or changes in relationships. None of these are easy battles, making effective coping strategies absolutely essential.

The current medical standard for treating depression in people with cancer is antidepressant medication and counseling. While medications may be somewhat successful, some patients do not respond well. Reasons for a lowered response include high stress and high levels of inflammation [1]. Low socioeconomic status, unemployment, poor working conditions, limited access to psychological services, and cultural attitudes toward medications may also reduce the efficacy of drugs [2]. Further, many cancer survivors are reluctant to take more medications because they fear the side effects of yet another pill.

For these reasons, complementary therapies are well-suited to assist. They are known to reduce stress, lower inflammation, and be accessible to everyone. These therapies have no adverse side effects and are acceptable across all cultures and backgrounds.

Complementary therapies for depression include various lifestyle changes, such as exercise, nutrition, and mind–body practices. Mind–body medicine is an integrative approach that focuses on the interconnectedness of the brain, mind, body, and behavior. It teaches coping techniques that promote self-awareness and self-care to support the mind's ability to influence our physical health, particularly for fatigue [3].

Let's explore how complementary therapies can support emotional wellness and help manage depression in people affected by cancer.

Complementary Treatments for Depression

Exercise

Exercise is one of the most evidence-based and practical tools for treating depression, and studies show it can be just as effective as antidepressant medications. Consequently, some are now suggesting that exercise become the new standard first-line therapy [4].

The link between exercise and depression works in both directions. First, people who are depressed are less likely to exercise. And second, people who don't exercise are more likely to become depressed. While it is noteworthy to point out this relationship, it matters not which came first. Recommending exercise to someone who states that they are depressed is an essential first step.

Both aerobic and resistance exercise are beneficial. Experts recommend 150 minutes per week of moderate to vigorous activity for protective effects against depression. Exercise has numerous positive effects, improving self-esteem, sleep quality, and overall quality of life, which in turn enhances mood and energy levels [5].

Still, it's important to acknowledge: mental health is complex. We all have a story and a past, and we all approach life's events differently. When we're feeling low, it's not easy to suddenly feel motivated and hopeful that exercising can lift the heaviness of our minds.

To make it more manageable, consider joining a prescheduled class or a community walking group. This eliminates the need to plan things yourself and gets you engaged with others. Pairing exercise with a positive environment also helps, such as going for a walk while listening to music or taking a bike ride in a park rather than down a busy street. Also, doing exercises that you enjoy is the key. If you find jogging boring, there's no need to force yourself to run. Try something new that feels good for your body.

And here's another helpful mindset shift: try thinking of physical activity as your daily medicine, just like a prescription. You need to take it for it to be effective and to make you feel better. Viewing exercise as your prescription will help you include it in your daily routine.

Yoga

Yoga aims to unify the body, mind, and spirit. This sense of integration can foster self-awareness, emotional balance, reduced stress, and great confidence. Multiple studies have shown that yoga is beneficial for those with depression, from mild symptoms of low mood to major depressive disorder [6]. It has been shown to reduce inflammation, lower stress hormones, and simultaneously increase our feel-good brain chemicals, including serotonin and dopamine [7].

If you're new to yoga, consider joining a beginner's class or trying various affordable apps. To help you get started, the following poses can support those with depression, as they are known as "heart openers," which involve opening up through the chest and hips. People experiencing depression often hold tension in these areas. By stretching these tight muscles, yoga can help release that physical tension and promote a feeling of openness and ease.

Only perform the poses that you are physically able to do and that won't cause strain on your neck, back, or knees. This is to give you an idea of some poses that can help, and you can modify the sequence as needed. Some poses are more advanced and may not be suitable for you, so feel free to skip them. Hold each pose for three breaths in and out, then gently transition to the next.

Suggested Yoga Sequence for Mood Support

1. Sphinx Pose—Lie on your stomach, then raise yourself onto your elbows. Keep your elbows aligned under your shoulders, and draw your shoulder blades back and down to open the chest.

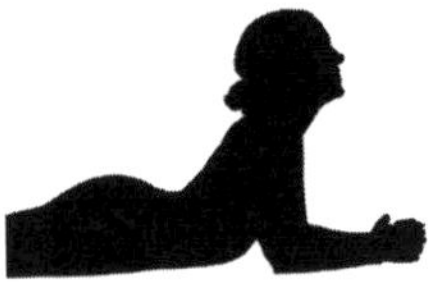

2. Cat/Cow Pose—Come onto your hands and knees. As you inhale, look up to the sky while dropping your belly, hold for a breath, and then, as you exhale, round your spine and focus your gaze on your belly.

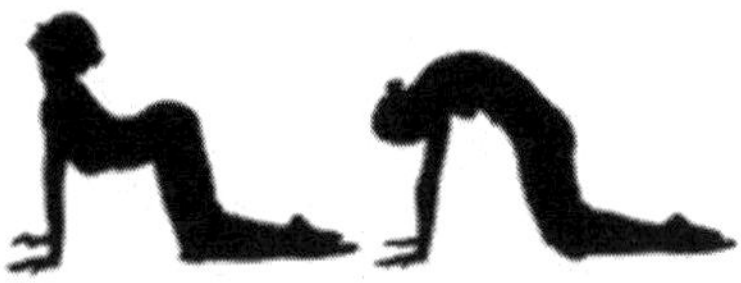

3. Puppy Pose—Return to all fours with a flat back, and while keeping your hips back, walk your hands forward and lower your forehead or chin to the ground, creating a long stretch through the spine and chest.

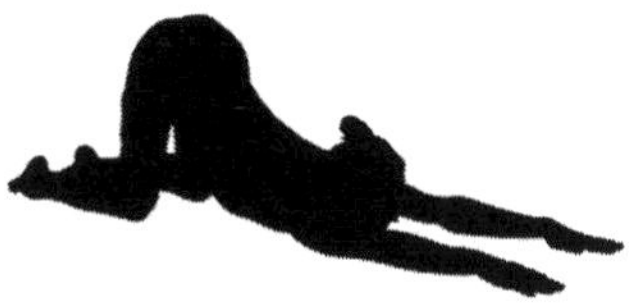

4. Bow Pose—This is an advanced move. Lie on your stomach, bend your knees, hold the outside of your ankles, and lift your chest.

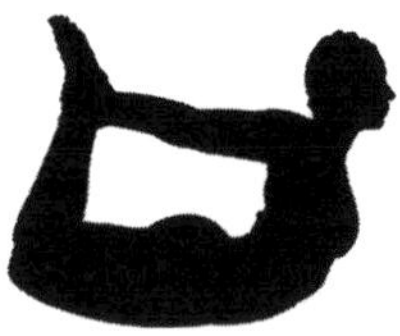

5. Fish Pose—This is an advanced pose. Lie on your back, bend your elbows, and lift your chest toward the sky. You can look up or bring the crown of your head to the floor.

6. Wheel Pose—This is an advanced move. Lie flat on your back, bend your knees, and place your hands beside your ears. Press into your palms and feet to lift your chest into a backbend.

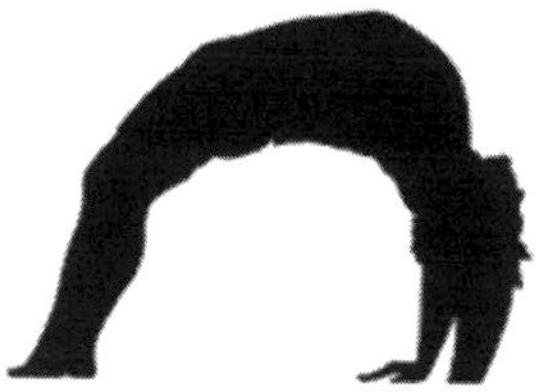

7. Crescent Lunge Pose—Transition into Downward Facing Dog pose, then bring one foot to the hand on the same side. Lower the opposite knee, lift your hands overhead, and deepen your stretch. Switch sides after two breaths.

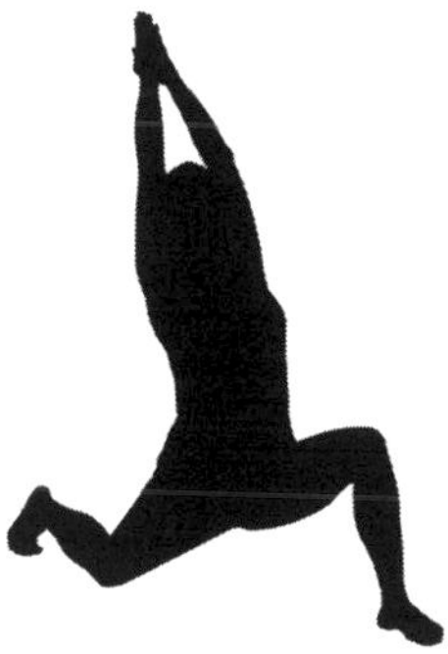

8. Reverse Warrior Pose—Stand up and move into Warrior 2 pose you learned earlier. Raise your front arm toward the sky and reach your back arm down the back of your leg. Switch sides after two breaths.

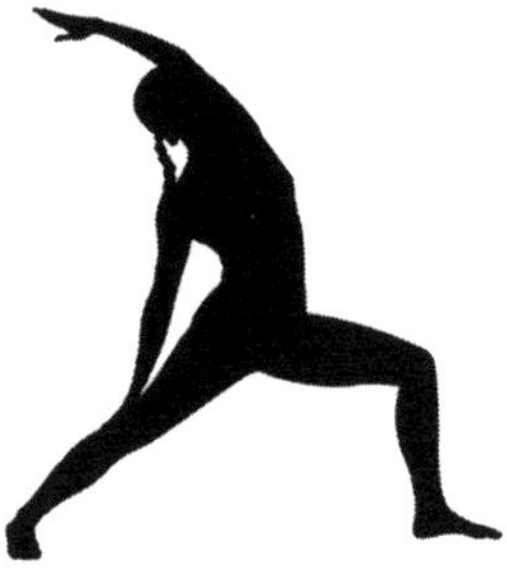

9. Dancer Pose—Stand upright, grasp the outside of your left foot with your left hand. Push your foot into your hand while bringing your other arm forward. Switch sides.

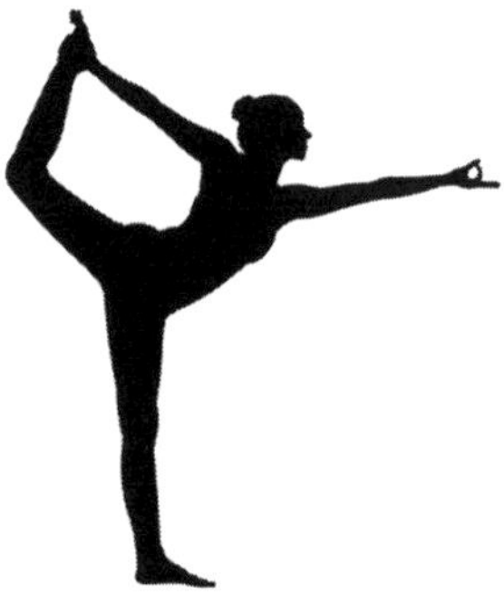

10. Standing Backbend Pose—Stand upright, push your hips forward, raise your arms overhead, and gently arch your upper back as you lift your chest toward the sky.

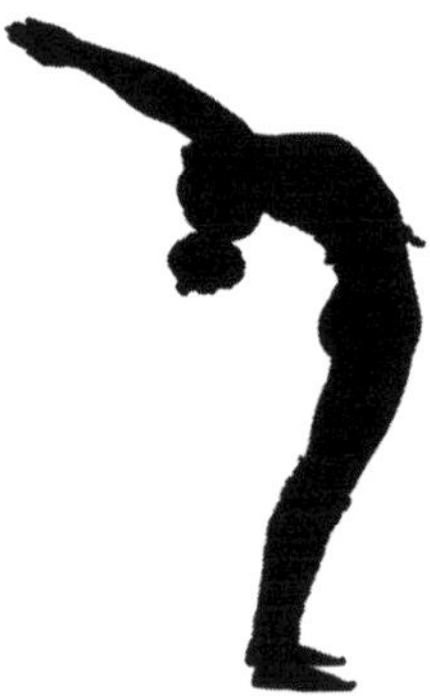

Mindfulness Meditation

Mindfulness meditation has been practiced for thousands of years, often as part of a spiritual practice. It can help reduce rumination, calm racing thoughts, and create space for greater acceptance and compassion, beneficial qualities when navigating depression after cancer. Research has found that meditation is highly effective for the treatment of depression [8] and for improving energy [9].

Meditation can be viewed as training your attention to achieve a state of calmness and foster positive emotions. What do you focus your attention on? The goal is to stay in the present moment by shifting your focus to your breath, thoughts, and physical sensations in your body.

For cancer survivors living with depression, this can help to cultivate a new perspective on themselves, consciously attend to the present moment, and approach new experiences with openness and acceptance [10]. When we turn our attention to the breath, we might notice we are holding it or breathing shallowly. We then mindfully incorporate breathing techniques, such as inhaling for five seconds and exhaling for five seconds, or even more slowly if you can.

Similarly, if we notice that our thoughts are filled with worry and rumination, we can remind ourselves to repeat the positive affirmations we've already created. If we feel physical tension, such as tight shoulders or a clenched jaw, we might pause and try a yoga pose to release it. Meditation ultimately links the mind and body, where one can positively influence the other.

Below is a guided meditation script designed to help you focus on your mood and energy.

This meditation is meant to create a gentle space for you to connect with yourself, recognize what you've been through, and cultivate a sense of calm and peaceful energy. You don't need to fix or change anything right now; allow yourself to be present.

Begin by finding a comfortable position, either sitting gently in a chair with your feet flat on the floor or lying down if that feels more supportive for your body. Allow your hands to rest gently in your lap or by your sides. If it feels comfortable, close your eyes or soften your gaze toward the floor.

Let's start by taking a few deep, intentional breaths. Inhale slowly through your nose, feeling your belly gently rise. And exhale slowly through your mouth, releasing any tension or thoughts that aren't serving you right now. Take another slow breath in... and out... allowing your body to settle a little more with each breath.

Now, allow your attention to rest on the natural rhythm of your breath. You don't need to change it or control it; just notice it. Feel the coolness of the air as it enters your nose... the slight expansion of your chest or belly... and the warm air leaving your body. Your breath is always here, a gentle anchor in the present moment.

As you continue to follow your breath, gently expand your awareness to include your entire body. Notice how your body feels right now at this moment. Without judgment, acknowledge any sensations present. You may notice areas of comfort... or areas of discomfort. There may be feelings of tiredness... or even moments of subtle energy. Whatever you notice, acknowledge it with kindness.

Now, let's focus on any thoughts or emotions that might be present, especially those related to fatigue or sadness. Visualize these thoughts and feelings as clouds moving across the sky. You don't need to hold onto them, analyze them, or push them away. Just notice them and then gently let them pass, making room for something new. It's all right for them to be there. This practice is about observing, not fixing.

If your mind wanders, which it naturally will, gently guide your attention back to your breath or the feeling of your body supported by the chair or the floor. Each time you bring your focus back, you're strengthening your ability to stay grounded with care and awareness.

Now, let's purposefully invite a gentle energy into your body. Visualize a soft, warm light starting to glow just behind your breastbone, at the center of your chest. This light signifies a subtle, peaceful energy.

With each inhale, picture this warm, gentle light expanding gradually, radiating outward to your shoulders, your arms, and your hands. Feel a soft, calming energy flowing through these areas.

With each exhale, release any remaining tension, making more room for this gentle energy to flow.

Now, with your next inhale, picture that light expanding downward through your torso... your hips... your legs... all the way to your feet. Let this calming warmth softly fill your body.

This isn't about feeling boundless energy, as you might have had before; it's about connecting with a quiet, sustainable energy that resides within you, even amidst exhaustion. Let this peaceful energy remind you of your resilience.

Hold onto this feeling of gentle energy and calm presence a little longer. Acknowledge yourself for taking this time to nourish your body and mind. You are giving yourself a valuable gift.

When you're ready to close the meditation, begin to deepen your breath. Feel the contact points of your body with the chair or the floor. Wiggle your fingers and toes, gently bringing movement back into your body.

And when you feel ready, open your eyes gently, taking this sense of peace and calm energy with you into the rest of your day. Remember, you can return to this practice whenever you need to reconnect with yourself. You are doing meaningful work by taking care of yourself.

Meditation's ability to boost energy levels can be understood not as creating energy out of nothing, but as retuning your being to access the underlying energy that already exists. It clears internal blocks and aligns you with the natural energy that sustains your body, mind, and spirit.

Fatigue often results from a misalignment between your physical body, emotional state, mental patterns, and spiritual essence. When your body feels tired but your mind cannot rest, or when your emotions become overwhelming but remain unprocessed, meditation helps create coherence and harmony among these different aspects of your being, leading to transformative experiences for some.

Worry, fear, constant mental chatter, and resisting the present moment are huge energy consumers. These are like "energy leaks" that drain your vitality. Meditation teaches you to observe these mental and emotional patterns without attachment, reducing their power to drain you. By cultivating presence and inner stillness, you plug these energetic leaks, allowing your energy to be retained and utilized more efficiently.

Meditation doesn't just manage symptoms; it facilitates a fundamental repatterning of your energetic self. It helps you become a clearer conduit for the universal energy that is always available, transforming fatigue into a deeper, more sustainable sense of vitality and presence.

Herbal Therapy

Plants contain potent compounds that interact with the body in ways that can enhance mood and reduce symptoms of depression. Some herbs can increase levels of serotonin, our "happy hormone," and enhance levels of GABA, which decrease feelings of stress. Others help improve sleep or protect the brain from inflammation. Numerous herbs may be helpful, but here are two that consistently improve depressive symptoms and have good research to back them up.

Saffron

The Latin name for this herb is *Crocus sativus*, and it is known for its use in Moroccan dishes due to its aroma, taste, and color. It has been shown to increase serotonin and dopamine levels in the brain, leading to an improved mood [11]. Multiple clinical trials have shown that Saffron is effective for improving the symptoms of mild, moderate, and severe depression [12]. Saffron also helps improve sleep, which helps immensely with depression [13].

CLINICAL PEARL

Begin with 15 mg twice daily for 12 weeks. If symptoms do not improve, consider increasing to 25 mg twice daily.

Rhodiola Rosea

Rhodiola has a strong reputation in traditional medicine. Over 140 distinct chemicals have been identified, which improve mood, memory, and energy, and reduce stress [14–16].

CLINICAL PEARL

Rhodiola doses typically range from 200 mg to 700 mg daily. Please start with the lowest dose to see how it works for you. If after eight weeks there is no improvement, increase the dose and assess how you feel.

Tai Chi

Research has shown that Tai chi can reduce depressive symptoms. Psychologically, these spiritual practices enhance well-being, self-esteem, self-awareness, and concentration, while also decreasing negative reactions and emotions [17].

Studies have shown that after practicing the movements, inflammation decreases, stress levels diminish, serotonin levels increase, and naturally occurring energy boosters, such as endorphins, are released [18]. Tai chi helps enhance internal peace and fosters a stronger connection between mind and body. It increases awareness of the surrounding environment, fosters self-growth, and can be very helpful for those struggling with depression.

Success Story

Fleur was diagnosed with bladder cancer, which required her bladder to be surgically removed. She was a yoga and dance teacher for many years and found it uncomfortable to resume her teaching after the placement of her urostomy pouch.

She developed a deep depression about her new circumstances and felt she didn't have a creative outlet anymore. She was also struggling with the new appearance of her body.

I suggested Tai Chi, as it can be viewed as a dance, and she could incorporate her own creative elements into it. I also explained how it could help with depression and maintain her physical fitness. She was interested and tried it.

One month later, she came to see me and was excited to share that she had found a new passion in Tai chi and was embarking on training to be able to teach and share this art with other cancer survivors who struggled with depression.

Nutrition

Throughout this book, we've emphasized the importance of nutrition as a key part of healing. Depression is no exception. Nutritional psychiatry is a growing field that investigates the link between diet and mental health, emphasizing how inflammation is a key factor. As nutritious foods possess anti-inflammatory properties, proper nutrition can support mental well-being.

Numerous studies have found that people who frequently choose nutritious whole foods are less likely to experience depression [19–21]. Mediterranean diets that focus on whole grains, fruits, vegetables, healthy fats, and lean proteins, while avoiding sugary foods, have been associated with lower rates of depression [22].

We can see convincing data indicating that changing our food choices can help improve our mood. This is also linked to the fact that eating better makes us feel like we are taking better care of ourselves, which naturally boosts our self-esteem and mood.

Lifestyle Psychiatry—Connectedness

Lifestyle psychiatry is an emerging field that focuses on preventing and treating mental health conditions through lifestyle changes like movement, sleep, nutrition, stress reduction, toxin avoidance, and social connection. Also referred to as lifestyle medicine, these types of recommendations are considered by many to be foundational components of mental health care.

We've already explored the benefits of movement and nutrition, and later chapters will address sleep and stress management. Toxic exposure reduction involves avoiding both environmental toxicants (polluted air, cigarette smoke, and alcohol) as well as social toxicants (social media, video games, and depressing news stories).

Connectedness is a unique concept that has not yet been discussed in this book, serving as a foundational element for addressing depression. It refers to the feeling of being part of something larger than yourself—feeling close to others, belonging to a group, and knowing you are seen, valued, and understood.

There are six domains of connectedness you can explore to better understand what may be missing from your life: happiness, purpose in life, empathy/compassion, social connection/community, nature, and spirituality/religion [23]. Let's consider these a bit further.

Happiness is a subjective concept, but it is primarily associated with experiencing joy often and feeling sad or angry less frequently. Interestingly, researchers have suggested that 50% of our happiness may be linked to our genes. This indicates that if you have a family history of depression, there is a strong likelihood that you might develop depression as well.

However, only 10% of happiness is attributed to external factors, such as money or marital status. That means a significant 40% comes from intentional actions—things we can deliberately do to boost our happiness [24]. So, try engaging in joyful activities daily to enhance your baseline happiness.

Finding purpose in life is also highly subjective and a lifelong quest, whether through work, setting and achieving goals, fulfilling specific family roles, or engaging in religious practices. Often, this puts us in contact with others who share a similar purpose, fostering a sense of connection.

Worth mentioning is the purpose found in work. Employment not only provides financial security but also significant psychological benefits. Being employed is a key source of personal identity, confidence, competence, social status, and self-esteem, and a lack of employment is associated with higher rates of depression [25]. Work also offers a daily schedule, which fosters a sense of routine and predictability. Of course, as long as job stress is not excessive, employment, even at reduced hours, can be very protective of mental health. For those who may not be able to work or are retired, volunteering offers similar benefits.

Empathy enables us to connect deeply with others, which helps build long-lasting relationships. Having empathy often allows us to feel compassion for others during difficult times. Strong, loving relationships founded on mutual empathy and compassion nurture a sense of social connection and deeper bonds.

The social impacts of living with depression can be extensive, potentially causing loneliness and isolation. When people isolate themselves, they may perceive their social support as worse, which can worsen depression and reduce energy levels. Staying connected, whether through religious groups, walking clubs, support circles, or hobbies, can offer structure, support, and hope.

Spending time in green spaces and nature also fosters a sense of connection and is a valuable lifestyle choice to consider. Whether it's a walk through a city park, caring for houseplants, or gardening in your backyard, nature reminds us of our place in the world and can offer calmness and renewal. Exposure to green spaces can help reduce depression by providing a positive outdoor environment with fresh air and a daily routine [26]. You might want to join a hiking group or take a horticulture class.

Connectedness is a protective factor, especially in the face of trauma. Having social support both during and after a cancer diagnosis is critical for long-term mental health, and therefore, connectedness is something that all cancer survivors should evaluate for themselves.

REFLECTION POINT—Begin to assess your sense of connectedness
1. Happiness—since 40% of your happiness is within your control, what activities do you find bring you joy? How frequently do you engage in these activities? Are you making time for them each day?

2. Sense of purpose—How do you feel about purpose? To what extent does employment or the lack of it influence your mood? Have you thought about volunteering?
3. Social connection—Are there any groups you've been wanting to join? A new hobby you'd like to try? Are there old friends you could reach out to for a weekly coffee meetup?
4. Nature—How often do you go outside? Are there parks nearby where you could take a daily walk? Do you have space in your yard to grow a small garden? Would you like to have more indoor plants?

Tapping

Also known as Emotional Freedom Technique (EFT), tapping is a mind–body therapy that is gaining recognition for its therapeutic value in addressing emotional concerns. What was once considered fringe "energy medicine" therapy is now supported by numerous clinical trials, and the evidence is promising. Tapping is also easy to learn, is free, and can be done anywhere, further empowering those with depression to feel more balanced and aid in their healing.

The technique involves gently tapping on specific acupressure points located on the head, face, and upper torso while repeating affirming statements. These affirmations are often phrased as statements of self-acceptance. For example, you might repeat, "Even though I'm not feeling my best, I fully love and accept myself." The theory is that by tapping on specific points, the area of the brain responsible for intense emotions is calmed, thereby diminishing the emotional intensity of particular thoughts or memories [27].

Tapping has measurable effects on the brain and body and has been shown to lower cortisol levels, increase serotonin, and decrease heart rate [28]. A recent meta-analysis looked at 18 randomized clinical trials and found that there was a substantial effect of tapping for depression [29].

CLINICAL PEARL

To try this out, follow these steps.

1. Identify a troubling issue or emotion. Rate how sad or upset you feel about it on a scale from 0 to 10—where 0 means no distress, and 10 is the most intense you've felt.
2. Create a statement that describes your issue, followed by a positive affirmation. For example, you could say, "Even though I feel sad that I'm not

working much at the moment, I am focusing on myself and am deeply committed to myself."

3. Tap repeatedly on the edge of your palm, below your little finger. While you tap, say your statement out loud three times.
4. Now tap on the rest of the points on your body, one at a time. While you tap, repeat your affirmation repeatedly.
5. The order of tapping is as follows: tap on the top center of your head, tap on the inside edge of one eyebrow, next tap the outside edge of one eye, then on the bone underneath one eye. Tap between your nose and your upper lip, between your lower lip and your chin, beneath one collarbone, and then under one armpit.
6. Stop and remeasure how you feel about your issue.
7. If needed, repeat the process. Tap until you can assign a lower number to your issue, or until you feel better.

Conclusion

The therapies explored in this chapter were chosen with care. All of these therapies encourage you to take good care of yourself. It is well understood that when individuals with depression adopt healthy lifestyle changes, they feel more connected to themselves and experience a strong sense of empowerment. As we conclude this chapter, you now hold essential knowledge to support recovery. The path ahead involves informed action, compassionate self-care, and unwavering hope. You can begin to restore your mind, re-energize your spirit, and embrace the vibrant life that lies ahead.

References

1 Miller AH, Maletic V, Raison CL. Inflammation and its discontents: the role of cytokines in the pathophysiology of major depression. Biol Psychiatry, 2009; 65(9):732–741.

2 Buckman JEJ, Saunders R, Stott J, et al. Socioeconomic indicators of treatment prognosis for adults with depression: a systematic review and individual patient data meta-analysis. JAMA Psychiatry, 2022; 79(5):406–416.

3 Astin JA, Shapiro SL, Eisenberg DM, et al. Mind-body medicine: state of the science, implications for practice. J Am Board Fam Pract, 2003; 16(2):131–147.

4 Heissel A, Heinen D, Brokmeier LL, et al. Exercise as medicine for depressive symptoms? A systematic review and meta-analysis with meta-regression. Br J Sports Med, 2023; 57(16):1049–1057.

5 Lederman O, Ward PB, Firth J, et al. Does exercise improve sleep quality in individuals with mental illness? A systematic review and meta-analysis. J Psych Res, 2019; 109:96–106.

6 Tolahunase MR, Sagar R, Faiq M, et al. Yoga- and meditation-based lifestyle intervention increases neuroplasticity and reduces severity of major depressive disorder: a randomized controlled trial. Restor Neurol Neurosci, 2018; 36(3):423–442.

7 Tolahunase MR, Gautam S, Sagar R, et al. Yoga in major depressive disorder: molecular mechanisms and clinical utility. Front Biosci Sch Ed, 2021; 13(1):56–81.

8 Huberty J, Puzia ME, Green J, et al. A mindfulness meditation mobile app improves depression and anxiety in adults with sleep disturbance: analysis from a randomized controlled trial. Gen Hosp Psychiatry, 2021; 73:30–37.

9 Park BJ, Choi Y, Lee JS, et al. Effectiveness of meditation for fatigue management: insight from a comprehensive systematic review and meta-analysis. Gen Hosp Psychiatry, 2024; 91:33–42.

10 Lamas-Morales P, Hijar-Aguinaga R, Garcia-Campayo J. Deconstructive meditations and psychotherapy: transforming the perception of the self. World J Psychiatry, 2025; 15(6):107505.

11 Matraszek-Gawron R, Chwil M, Terlecki K, et al. Current knowledge of the antidepressant activity of chemical compounds from *Crocus sativus* L. Pharm (Basel Switzerland), 2022; 16:58.

12 Siddiqui SA, Ali Redha A, Snoeck ER, et al. Anti-depressant properties of crocin molecules in saffron. Mol (Basel Switzerland), 2022; 27:2076.

13 Munirah MP, Norhayati MN, Noraini M. Crocus sativus for insomnia: a systematic review and meta-analysis. Int J Environ Res Public Health, 2022; 19:11658.

14 Mao JJ, Xie SX, Zee J, et al. Rhodiola rosea versus sertraline for major depressive disorder: a randomized placebo-controlled trial. Phytomedicine, 2015; 22:394–399.

15 Gao L, Wu C, Liao Y, et al. Antidepressants effects of Rhodiola capsule combined with sertraline for major depressive disorder: a randomized double-blind placebo-controlled clinical trial. J Affect Disord, 2020; 265:99–103.

16 European Medicines Agency. Committee on Herbal Medicinal Products (HMPC) Assessment Report on *Rhodiola rosea* L., Rhizoma Et Radix. European Medicines Agency; Amsterdam, The Netherlands: 2011. Document Reference. EMA/HMPC/232100/2011.

17 Easwaran K, Gopalasingam Y, Green DD, et al. Effectiveness of Tai Chi for health promotion for adults with health conditions: a scoping review of meta-analyses. Disabil Rehabil, 2021; 43(21):2978–2989.

18 Lu EY, Lee P, Cai S, et al. Qigong for the treatment of depressive symptoms: preliminary evidence of neurobiological mechanisms. Int J Geriatr Psychiatry, 2020; 35(11):1393–1401.

19 Cebrino J, de la Cruz SP. Quality and sociodemographic, lifestyle, and health-related determinants among people with depression in Spain: new evidence from a cross-sectional population-based study. Nutrients, 2020; 13(1):106.
20 Molendijk M, Molero P, Ortuño Sánchez-Pedreño F, et al. Diet quality and depression risk: a systematic review and dose-response meta-analysis of prospective studies. J Affect Disord, 2018; 226:346–354.
21 Lassale C, Batty GD, Baghdadli A, et al. Healthy dietary indices and risk of depressive outcomes: a systematic review and meta-analysis of observational studies. Mol Psychiatry, 2019; 24:965–986.
22 Jacka FN, O'Neil A, Opie R, et al. Randomized controlled trial of dietary improvement for adults with major depression (the 'SMILES' trial). BMC Med, 2017; 15:23.
23 Merlo G, Snellman L, Sugden SG. Connectedness: the updated and expanded pillar of lifestyle psychiatry and lifestyle medicine. Am J Lifestyle Med, 2025; 15598276251345455.
24 Lyubomirsky S, Sheldon KM, Schkade D. Pursuing happiness: the architecture of sustainable change. Rev Gen Psychol, 2005; 9(2):111–131.
25 van der Noordt M, Ijzelenberg H, Droomers M, et al. Health effects of employment: a systematic review of prospective studies. Occupational Environmental Medicine, 2014; 71(10):730–736.
26 Masterton W, Carver H, Parkes T, et al. Greenspace interventions for mental health in clinical and non-clinical populations: What works, for whom, and in what circumstances? Health Place, 2020; 64:102338.
27 Church D, David I. Borrowing benefits: clinical EFT (emotional freedom techniques) as an immediate stress reduction skill in the workplace. Psychology, 2019; 10:941–952.
28 Church D, Yount G, Brooks AJ. The effect of emotional freedom techniques on stress biochemistry: a randomized controlled trial. J Nerv Ment Dis, 2012; 200:891–896.
29 Seok JW, Kim JU. The effectiveness of emotional freedom techniques for depressive symptoms: a meta-analysis. J Clin Med, 2024; 13(21):6481.

12

The Stress and Anxiety Reset

> *Our anxiety does not empty tomorrow of its sorrows, But only today, of its strengths*
>
> —C.H. Sturgeon

> *Sometimes the most important thing in a whole day is the rest we take between two deep breaths*
>
> —Etty Hillesum

This chapter is for you if:

- You've noticed that anxiety is a familiar part of your life, and cancer has only heightened it.
- You're living with a high level of stress and feel unequipped to manage it.
- You have a high level of stress and wonder how this might be negatively affecting you.
- You are currently on antianxiety medication and are curious about other supportive therapies.

Stress and Distress

While the physical toll of cancer is undeniable, the invisible burdens of anxiety and stress can also profoundly drain your energy, making that persistent cancer-related fatigue (CRF) feel even heavier. It's easy to overlook the significant impact our thoughts and worries have on our physical well-being. This chapter is dedicated to showing you how, by gently addressing anxiety and stress, you can

Beyond Cancer Fatigue: A Path to Reclaiming Energy, First Edition. Jessa Landmann, ND.

unlock a surprising reserve of energy and embrace a more peaceful and energetic life.

Think of chronic stress as a leaky faucet. Just as the steady drip wastes water, the persistent drip of stress slowly depletes our energy. A potentially life-threatening illness like cancer is understandably one of the most stressful experiences in a person's life. There is stress and worry about one's prognosis, what the treatments might be like, worries about family members, and what the future might hold.

While our bodies are incredibly equipped with a "fight or flight" response for short bursts of pressure—whether it's navigating a crowd, fighting a cold, or dealing with a difficult person—cancer isn't a short-term stressor that simply comes and goes.

This is where the power of your mind comes in. It can be your greatest ally or your biggest obstacle. When our thoughts and emotions related to cancer remain unresolved, stress can linger long after the initial shock, pushing us into a chronic state of distress. But by recognizing this powerful connection, we can begin to learn how to turn down that faucet and preserve the energy you need for healing and living.

Distress is often regarded as the "sixth vital sign." Vital signs measure crucial physiological functions, including body temperature, pulse rate, blood pressure, respiratory rate, and the presence of pain. These measurements are routinely taken during medical visits. But when was the last time someone asked how distressed you felt?

The National Comprehensive Cancer Network defines distress as "a multifactorial unpleasant emotional experience of a psychological, social, and/or spiritual nature that may interfere with the ability to cope effectively with cancer, its physical symptoms, and its treatment. Distress extends along a continuum, from common normal feelings of vulnerability, sadness, and fears to problems that can become disabling, such as depression, anxiety, panic, social isolation, and existential spiritual crisis."

Imagine if we treated emotional well-being with the same urgency as a fever or high blood pressure. This is the powerful idea behind recognizing distress as a "sixth vital sign" in cancer care. It underscores just how crucial your emotional health is, not just for your quality of life, but for your overall well-being and even your journey toward healing. While it's entirely natural for every patient to experience some level of distress after a cancer diagnosis, about one-third will encounter a depth of distress that genuinely needs specific support [1].

Screening for distress is essential because it's linked to fatigue, anxiety, poor sleep, and a poorer quality of life. It's a two-way street: fatigue can worsen distress, and distress, in turn, can intensify fatigue [2]. By actively managing stress, you initiate a powerful, positive cycle that helps alleviate your overall burden, foster your resilience, and enhance your energy.

Anxiety

Closely linked to stress and distress is anxiety, which is a feeling of fear, dread, or unease about something immediate or something yet to come. The perceived threats can be both real and imagined. Physical symptoms that may occur as a result of anxiety include increased heart rate, muscle tension, insomnia, and fatigue.

People who have gone through cancer often tend to have higher anxiety levels than the general population. One study found that about 35% of women with breast cancer experienced anxiety, a rate three times greater than those without a cancer diagnosis [3]. The more severe their anxiety, the more severe their fatigue tended to be.

The same is true for survivors of colon cancer. Prevalence rates of anxiety in that group are as high as 50% [4], which correlates with the prevalence rate of fatigue in that population, also at 50% [5].

Stress and anxiety significantly contribute to CRF, primarily due to one key player: cortisol. Cortisol is our primary stress hormone, and while it is a hormone we cannot live without, when it is consistently elevated, it wreaks havoc on our bodies.

Understanding Stress/Anxiety and Fatigue

As you've learned, when faced with a state of stress and anxiety, your body naturally activates its "fight or flight" response, which triggers a rapid release of cortisol, preparing you for immediate action with a surging heart rate, tense muscles, and a quick surge in blood sugar. In short bursts, such as escaping danger, these changes are beneficial, allowing you to react swiftly and effectively.

However, the challenge arises when stress becomes a constant companion, as it often does during and after a cancer diagnosis. Unlike a fleeting threat, ongoing worries result in a persistent elevation of cortisol, which has significant consequences for your energy levels.

Cortisol keeps us on high alert, and this relentless demand can leave you feeling drained and exhausted. Cortisol also contributes to fatigue by breaking down muscle tissue, leading to physical weakness. As we will discuss in Chapter 14, this elevated cortisol disrupts your natural sleep–wake cycle, making it harder to get restorative rest and intensifying daytime fatigue. Furthermore, a prolonged stress response can suppress neurotransmitters that elevate our mood, such as serotonin and dopamine, which can contribute to feelings of low energy and fatigue.

The influence of stress goes beyond hormonal imbalances. It can significantly reduce your appetite, affecting your ability to nourish your body and maintain vital energy. Stress also impacts digestion, possibly blocking nutrient absorption when you eat. The persistent muscle tension and headaches contribute to your overall fatigue. And perhaps most insidiously, the mental burden of chronic worry is incredibly draining. Even if you seem strong outwardly, an internal "emotional tornado" of stress can quietly drain your energy, day after day.

There's no quick fix for deeply ingrained stress. It requires a journey of self-awareness and self-compassion. In the following sections, we'll explore practical strategies to help you navigate and effectively manage these emotions, ultimately empowering you to reclaim your energy and improve your quality of life.

REFLECTION POINT

Are you experiencing any physical symptoms of high cortisol? Do you notice changes in your appetite, sleep problems, irritability, or muscle pain? These could be signs that you are in a state of stress, and managing stress can significantly improve your physical well-being. Are you unsure if you're in distress and might need extra support? Revisit the definition of distress and see if it resonates with you.

Treatments for Stress and Anxiety

Practicing Self-awareness and Mindfulness

Self-awareness is a fundamental skill that significantly helps to reduce stress and anxiety by empowering us to understand, interpret, and respond to our internal and external experiences more effectively. It involves tuning into your thoughts, emotions, physical sensations, and behaviors, without judgment. This concept is similar to mindfulness.

Self-awareness begins with understanding what triggers your stress. When you're self-aware, you can start to notice patterns in what causes you stress or anxiety. Is it a particular person, a type of task, a specific environment, or even certain thoughts? By recognizing these triggers, you gain valuable information that allows you to avoid them, prepare for them, or develop strategies to cope with them when they arise. Without self-awareness, everything can feel overwhelming, and you may feel helpless.

Self-awareness enables you to name emotions as they arise. Instead of being consumed by a wave of "bad feelings," you can recognize if it's anxiety, anger, frustration, sadness, or something else. The simple act of naming an emotion can create a sense of distance and control, reducing its intensity. Consider using a "feeling wheel" as a tool; it offers a broader vocabulary for emotions, helping you articulate what you're feeling more clearly.

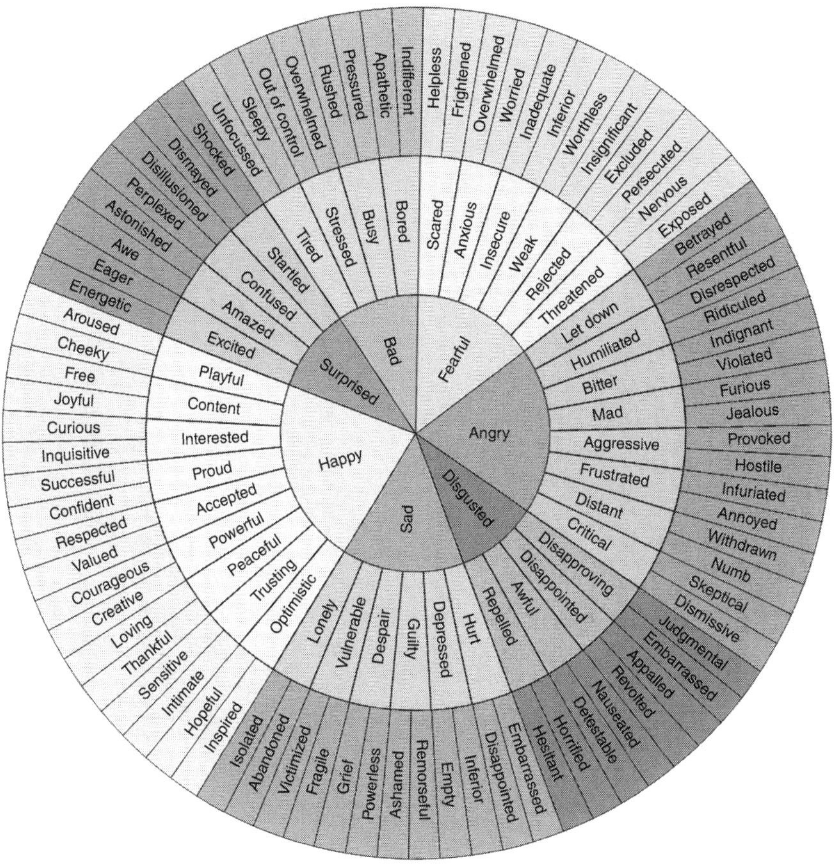

When you're self-aware, you move from reacting impulsively to responding thoughtfully. You can pause, acknowledge your emotions, and then consciously decide how to act. For instance, if you recognize you felt dismissed in an appointment, you can write out and practice how you want to communicate that you need more time to ask questions. Self-awareness may also prompt you to take a short break, re-prioritize, or ask for help, instead of spiraling into panic or frustration.

Anxiety often involves rumination—getting stuck in repetitive negative thoughts about the past or future. Self-awareness enables you to recognize yourself in this loop and provides the opportunity to gently redirect your attention to the present moment or engage in constructive problem-solving.

Self-awareness involves understanding your strengths and limitations, recognizing your energy patterns, and learning what you need to thrive. This enables you to set healthy boundaries, say "no" to commitments that would overwhelm you, and prioritize self-care activities (like sleep, exercise, or relaxation) that genuinely replenish you.

In essence, self-awareness acts as an internal compass and an early warning system. It provides the foundation for choice and control, empowering you to navigate life's challenges with greater clarity, resilience, and intentionality, ultimately leading to a significant reduction in stress and anxiety.

REFLECTION POINT

Make a list of the situations that cause you the most stress and anxiety. It could be upcoming appointments, a work colleague you don't get along with, or a lingering pain you can't figure out. Perhaps you find weekly grocery shopping stressful, or you've overcommitted to projects you don't care about.

Can you avoid any of your stressors? If not, how can you manage them when they arise? Do you struggle to say no to others? Practice phrases like "let me get back to you," instead of agreeing immediately. Are you making time for self-care? Do you exercise, spend time outdoors in nature, or dedicate time to your hobbies? Schedule moments for relaxation.

Practice using the feelings wheel to find new words for emotions you often feel. This can help you recognize feelings in the moment, which can lessen your stress.

Herbal Treatments for Anxiety

Ashwagandha

Ashwagandha has been used since 6,000 BC, making it one of the oldest known medicinal herbs. It possesses anti-inflammatory, antioxidant, anticancer, immune-stimulating, antidepressant, and antianxiety properties [6].

Ashwagandha can effectively reduce anxiety in adults with generalized anxiety disorder [7]. The reason for this is that Ashwagandha lowers cortisol levels. One study observed a 41% reduction in anxiety scores and a 23% decrease in morning cortisol levels after 60 days of taking Ashwagandha daily [8]. Additionally, serotonin levels are increased, improving depression, anxiety, and sleep [9]. Due to its cortisol-lowering properties, Ashwagandha improves sleep in those struggling with insomnia [10].

CLINICAL PEARL

Ashwagandha is my go-to for stress and anxiety. It effectively reduces cortisol, helps with mood issues like anxiety and depression, and tends to enhance sleep and energy. Begin with 250 mg three times daily.

Success Story

Ming was diagnosed with ovarian cancer and was successfully treated with surgery and chemotherapy. She had read a lot about how aggressive ovarian cancer can be, and she constantly worried about her well-being. She worried about caring for her husband and her elderly mother. She used to be very active in group exercise classes but hadn't resumed those activities yet. She also worried that she wasn't exercising!

Ming told me she couldn't stop crying. She said she cried all day long and couldn't stop even if she tried. She mentioned her anxiety was a 10/10 and that she was having trouble sleeping and focusing. I suggested Ashwagandha to reduce her anxiety and help her cope.

Two weeks later, she said her anxiety was at a 5/10, and she felt more balanced. We explored the feelings wheel, and instead of sadness, she identified feeling embarrassed and ashamed. She realized she didn't want to return to the exercise classes because she had lost her hair, and she felt embarrassed that she was "sick."

Ming always considered herself a healthy person, and she was ashamed that she got cancer despite her best efforts. Once she identified the root of her crying, she cried less often. She did some further counseling, and after realizing that cancer was not her fault, she felt less ashamed and returned to her old classes, reuniting with supportive friends. She felt Ashwagandha enabled her to reduce her emotional intensity and be more self-aware.

Lavender

Lavender is not only a beautiful plant to look at, but it has also been used for centuries for its calming effects. Its folkloric reputation has since been supported by scientific research, as lavender has been found to help alleviate anxiety in various populations. The effects of lavender are due to its essential oil content, and it can be used through aromatherapy or oral supplements. Lavender has been found to slow the heart rate, slow breathing, lower blood pressure, reduce cortisol levels, and act on the brain centers that promote relaxation [11].

Lavender has been shown to reduce anxiety in many settings: it calms people before dental work, it lessens anxiety before an MRI, and it lessens anxiety before a bone marrow biopsy [12]. In some cases, its effects are comparable to prescription antianxiety medications [13].

CLINICAL PEARL

Lavender would be my second choice for anxiety if Ashwagandha were not effective. For aromatherapy, try adding 20 drops of essential oil to 250 ml of water or 10 drops to 100 ml of water. You can keep the diffuser in your car, at work, or anywhere in your home. Oral lavender supplements are also suitable. Start with 80 mg twice daily.

Exercise

Boxing

Just like depression, exercise is highly recommended for stress and anxiety as well. Both aerobic exercise and weight lifting, as well as relaxing forms of activity such as yoga, are beneficial in lowering stress. But given that people with stress and anxiety often feel quite tense and need a physical release, this section will draw attention to one specific form of exercise: boxing. If you are a patient of mine, you are likely chuckling to yourself, as this is something that is often recommended to my patients.

What you need to understand is that the recommendation here is not for competitive boxing against an opponent, where injury or pain could happen. The type of boxing we're discussing is for stress relief, fitness, and fun. Boxing gyms are appearing all around the world, as it is recognized as a great way to manage stress. These gyms often involve working with a heavy bag or with someone holding pads. However, if an organized boxing class isn't accessible or affordable, shadowboxing—a form of boxing where you punch the air—is just as effective.

Concerning mental health, 94% of studies have found that boxing improves mood, reduces substance use, elevates self-esteem and confidence, enhances one's perception of physical ability, and improves overall health and well-being [14]. Boxing is an effective way to alleviate anger and can be helpful even for those who have experienced traumatic events, such as a cancer diagnosis [15].

Breathing Techniques

The way we breathe profoundly impacts our body's stress response, and while it may seem like a small detail, intentionally slowing and deepening your breath, primarily through your nose, can calm your nervous system and reduce anxiety.

When we breathe through the mouth, our breaths tend to be quicker and shallower. This faster breathing can trigger the "fight or flight" response in the brain, making us feel more stressed. When we breathe through the nose, breaths are slower and deeper, which activates the calming parts of our brain and reduces feelings of stress and anxiety.

Slow breathing at a rate of four to six breaths per minute activates our vagus nerve, slows the heart rate, and even slows brain waves [16]. These changes support clearer thinking, better sleep, less anxiety, and more stable energy.

Throughout the book, you've learned about mindfulness through mindful walking or meditation. During these practices, deep breathing is incorporated and helps slow the mind. During yoga, breathing is slowed and timed with movement. Deep breathing is also discussed in Chapter 14. These moments are opportunities to anchor your awareness to your breath.

There are many breathing techniques you can try. One popular method is called box breathing. This involves inhaling for four seconds, holding it for four seconds, exhaling for four seconds, and then holding it again for four seconds. This results in four breaths per minute and is highly effective for calming the mind. There's no perfect method; choose what feels natural and grounding to you.

Other Stress Management Techniques

When it comes to stress management, it is highly personal. You may feel grounded during mindfulness practice. Or you may enjoy listening to music. Or perhaps you like to knit. You may want to take up gardening. Or maybe you're exploring the art of writing poetry. It does not matter. What matters is that you take steps to manage your stress.

Many types of stress management therapies have been explored for cancer survivors. Art therapy is an intriguing field, and all kinds of art have been studied, including painting with watercolors, drawing, and even working with clay. Art therapy has also been found to be helpful for caregivers helping their loved ones with cancer [17].

Singing is another powerful tool found to reduce stress and lower anxiety in people with cancer and their family members. One study examined the benefits of joining a choir and found that cortisol levels decreased and feelings of connectedness improved [18].

The most important message is this: find something that feels meaningful and enjoyable, and make space for it in your life, most days of the week.

Conclusion

It is natural to feel stressed out. It is normal to feel angry and overwhelmed, or sad. However, the problem arises when these feelings persist unchecked, as they can take over one's life. We previously discussed self-awareness and mindfulness, and this is the stepping stone to 1) identifying our emotions and then 2) engaging in activities that can help to reduce the intensity of those emotions.

By actively addressing these psychological burdens, patients can interrupt the vicious cycle where emotional distress exacerbates fatigue. This opens the door to improved energy, greater emotional resilience, and a renewed ability to engage with life on their terms. Ultimately, cultivating strategies for emotional regulation and stress reduction empowers those with CRF to reclaim a sense of control, foster resilience, and significantly elevate their overall well-being and quality of life throughout their cancer journey.

References

1 Bultz BD, Carlson LE. Emotional distress: the sixth vital sign in cancer care. J Clin Oncol, 2005; 23:6440–6441.
2 Stepanski EJ, Walker MS, Schwatrzberg LS, et al. The relation of trouble sleeping, depressed mood, pain and fatigue in patients with cancer. J Clin Sleep Med, 2009; 5:132–136.
3 Williams AM, Khan CP, Heckler CE, et al. Fatigue, anxiety and quality of life in breast cancer patients compared to non-cancer controls: a nationwide longitudinal analysis. Breast Cancer Res Treat, 2022; 187(1):275–285.
4 Peng YN, Huang ML, Kao CH. Prevalence of depression and anxiety in colorectal cancer patients: a literature review. Int J Environ Res Publ Health, 2019; 16(3):411.
5 Walling AM, Weeks JC, Kahn KL, et al. Symptom prevalence in lung and colorectal cancer patients. J Pain Symptom Manag, 2015; 49(2):192–202.
6 Bhattacharya SK, Bhattacharya A, Sairam K, et al. Anxiolytic-antidepressant activity of Withania somnifera glycowithanolides: an experimental study. Phytomedicine, 2000; 7:463–469.
7 Andrade C, Aswath A, Chaturvedi SK, et al. A double-blind, placebo-controlled evaluation of the anxiolytic efficacy of an ethanolic extract of *Withania somnifera*. Indian J Psychiatry, 2000; 42:295–301.
8 Lopresti AL, Smith SJ, Malvi H, et al. An investigation into the stress-relieving and pharmacological actions of an ashwaghanda (*Withania somnifera*) extract. Medicine, 2019; 98(37):e17186.

9 Majeed M, Nagabhushanam K, Murali A, et al. A standardized *Withania somnifera* (Linn.) root extract with pipeline alleviates the symptoms of anxiety and depression by increasing serotonin levels: a double-blind randomized placebo-controlled study. J Integer Complement Med, 2024; 30(5):459–468.

10 Langade D, Thakare V, Kanchi S, et al. Clinical evaluation of the pharmacological impact of ashwaghanda root extract on sleep in healthy volunteers and insomnia patients: a double-blind randomized parallel-group, placebo-controlled study. J Ethnopharmacol, 2021; 264:113276.

11 Kang HJ, Nam ES, Lee Y, et al. How strong is the evidence for the anxiolytic efficacy of lavender?: a systematic review and meta-analysis of randomized controlled trials. Asian Nurs Res, 2019; 13(5):295–305.

12 Abbaszadeh R, Tabari F, Asadpour A. The effect of lavender aroma on anxiety of patients having bone marrow biopsy. Asian Pac J Cancer Prev, 2020; 21(3):771–775.

13 Woelk H, Schalke S. A multi-center, double-blind, randomized study of lavender oil preparation Silexan in comparison to Lorazepam for generalized anxiety disorder. Phytomedicine, 2010; 17(2):94–99.

14 Bozdarov J, Jones BDM, Daskalakis ZJ, et al. Boxing as an intervention in mental health: a scoping review. Am J Lifestyle Med, 2022; 17(4):589–600.

15 Gammage KL, van Ingen C, Angrish K. Measuring the effects of the shape your life project on the mental and physical health outcomes of survivors of gender-based violence. Violence Against Women, 2021; 28:2722–2741.

16 Tang YY, Tang R, Rothbart MK, et al. Frontal theta activity and white matter plasticity following mindfulness meditation. Curr Opin Psychol, 2019; 10:1016.

17 Zhang M, Liu X, Huang Y. Are art-based interventions effective in improving psychological well-being among informal caregivers of cancer patients? A systematic review. J Integr Complement Med, 2025; 31(1):11–24.

18 Fancourt D, Williamon A, Carvalho LA, et al. Singing modulates mood, stress, cortisol, cytokine and neuropeptide activity in cancer patients and carers. Ecancermedicalscience, 2016; 10:631.

13

Living Fully Despite Fear of Recurrence

Inaction breeds doubt and fear. Action breeds confidence and courage. If you want to conquer fear, do not sit home and think about it. Go out and get busy

—Dale Carnegie

This chapter is for you if:

- You've overcome cancer but struggle with intrusive thoughts about recurrence.
- You would like proactive strategies for dealing with fears and worries about a cancer recurrence.

For countless cancer survivors, the journey beyond treatment often brings a pervasive and profound challenge: the fear of cancer recurrence (FCR). This isn't just a fleeting worry, but an intense, ongoing preoccupation, where every ache or new sensation can be misinterpreted as a grim sign that cancer has returned. While this fear can naturally subside over time, for many it lingers, casting a long shadow over their hard-won sense of well-being.

This constant vigilance, coupled with a tendency toward rumination—those relentless, negative thought loops about what might go wrong—directly fuels a cycle of emotional distress, making that already challenging cancer-related fatigue feel even heavier [1].

The connection between your physical symptoms and your deepest fears cannot be overstated. Studies show that sensations like pain and fatigue are most often misinterpreted as ominous signs of recurrence, creating a direct pathway where physical discomfort escalates into psychological distress [2]. This relationship is bidirectional, though—fatigue can lead to fear of recurrence, but fear of recurrence can also lead to fatigue, creating a "chicken and egg" situation about what came first. So where do we start?

Beyond Cancer Fatigue: A Path to Reclaiming Energy, First Edition. Jessa Landmann, ND.

There's compelling evidence that improving your energy levels can be a powerful first step in alleviating the fear of recurrence. Imagine the relief of breaking free from the constant internal alarm, allowing your body and mind to truly rest and recover. By proactively addressing fatigue, you're not only improving a physical symptom but also directly impacting your mental peace and emotional resilience.

How do you improve energy? By addressing any of the factors contributing to fatigue in this book! Focus on nutrition, exercise, sleep, and stress management. Reduce other nagging issues, such as pain or hot flashes. Throughout this book, you've been discovering for yourself what the biggest and most significant sources of your energy drain are.

However, fear of recurrence also arises from other factors, such as "scanxiety" (anxiety about upcoming imaging appointments), media stories, anniversaries of diagnoses, trauma from treatments, or the dreaded prognosis statistics. These intense fears can then lead to fatigue. This presents a nuanced perspective on the relationship between fatigue and the fear of recurrence. This cycle must be broken, and you have the power to influence it.

By recognizing the link between fear and fatigue, you can start to dismantle this challenging loop. This chapter will guide you through practical, empowering strategies to manage both your energy and your fears, paving the way for a life lived more fully in the present, with a renewed sense of hope and peace.

How to Lessen Fears of Cancer Recurrence

Health Behavior Change

A recent survey found that less than 10% of cancer survivors follow lifestyle guidelines known to reduce recurrence [3]. Those who don't follow these recommendations often experience a heightened fear of recurrence [4]. Patients may not be informed about the numerous lifestyle changes that can significantly impact their lives.

Therefore, it is the strong recommendation of this book that every cancer survivor should be educated, as part of the standard of medical care, on how lifestyle improvements can lower their risk of cancer recurrence, as this will directly translate into less fear of its return.

Nutrition guidelines recommend a high intake of fruits and vegetables and a low intake of added sugars, as these are associated with a statistically significant reduction in cancer recurrence [5]. Adherence to a Mediterranean diet has consistently been shown to reduce the risk of disease recurrence [6]. A lower consumption of red meat, which includes beef, pork, and lamb, is linked with reduced risk of recurrence. Higher fiber intake and higher soy intake [7] are connected to lower recurrence rates, particularly in survivors of breast cancer.

What we know about physical activity and cancer recurrence is also clear: a greater amount of physical activity is associated with a reduced risk of cancer recurrence [8]. Exercise reduces inflammation, boosts mood, improves sleep, lowers blood sugar, and aids in weight control, all key factors in preventing recurrence.

Sleep is also associated with cancer recurrence rates, as you'll read in Chapter 14. Both oversleeping (more than nine hours per night) and sleep deprivation (less than five hours per night) have been linked to increased risk of recurrence in survivors of colon cancer [8].

Both smoking cessation and reducing alcohol intake reduce recurrence rates and improve survival as well [8].

One potential obstacle getting in the way of health behavior change is the lack of belief that lifestyle changes can help reduce recurrence. It's easy to feel as if our daily choices don't matter when it comes to health, especially after a cancer diagnosis. Perhaps you've thought, "What's the point of making big lifestyle changes if cancer can still strike anyone?" We've all known someone who seemed to do everything "right"—eating perfectly, exercising regularly, living a joyful life—only to still receive the unsettling news of a cancer diagnosis. This can lead to a sense of helplessness, making it hard to believe that our efforts truly make a difference in reducing the risk of recurrence.

Here's a powerful truth: it's estimated that a remarkable 45–70% of cancers could potentially be prevented by focusing on lifestyle factors. This isn't about fate; it's about empowerment. Factors like our diet, exercise habits, alcohol consumption, and whether we smoke hold incredible sway over our health destiny.

This is a call to action. This information should be shared across social media, and these facts should be repeated in our conversations with doctors and other loved ones. The more visibly and consistently this life-saving information is presented, the more deeply it will resonate, becoming not just credible but truly impactful. The impact it will make is on lessening the fear of recurrence so that cancer survivors can live a life not handcuffed to these daily worries.

Health behavior change is most likely to succeed when internal motivation is strong. To foster this, take small steps, keep things interesting, and practice positive self-talk. For example, when trying to incorporate exercise into your routine, you will be more motivated if you start with small steps, such as walking for 10 minutes each day, instead of attempting a 5-km run. To incorporate more fruits and vegetables into your diet, try learning five new recipes to mix things up and avoid eating the same thing every day. This way, your food stays interesting and varied.

We need to remember that every small decision counts in the long run. Think of your health like building a house—it doesn't look like much when we only lay the foundation, but we keep going because eventually, we have protective walls and a solid roof over our heads. We should remind ourselves of this every day and use positive, encouraging language to remind ourselves that what we are doing truly makes a difference.

REFLECTION POINT

Were you aware of lifestyle changes that can reduce the risk of recurrence? Do you feel you are following the guidelines regarding nutrition, sleep, exercise, smoking, and alcohol? If not, do you think that following the guidelines would help you feel less fear?

Do you believe that your efforts to prevent cancer make a difference? Why or why not? If not, review the chapters on nutrition, diabetes, weight management, and sleep.

If you don't follow guidelines for lifestyle changes, what small steps could you take today?

Post-traumatic Growth

Over the past few decades, significant improvements in cancer treatments have led to a considerable rise in survival rates. However, as we discussed earlier in this book, many survivors continue to face ongoing challenges such as fatigue, low mood, poor sleep, cognitive issues, and a reduced quality of life long after their treatment has ended.

Survivors also carry physical and emotional scars from their treatments, such as disfiguring surgeries and painful procedures. They have frightening memories and feel uncertain about what lies ahead. With these burdens in mind, it's understandable that moving forward can feel daunting.

One effective way to cope is by reframing how we view such a transformative event, possibly turning a negative experience into a springboard for positive growth. Indeed, positive psychological changes can result from struggling against a frightening life event, a process known as post-traumatic growth (PTG). PTG refers to the positive shifts that can occur when navigating highly stressful situations. PTG is associated with an improved quality of life, reduced distress, and a more positive outlook [9].

This growth can appear as a greater appreciation for life, stronger connections with others, a heightened sense of personal strength, and the development of new possibilities. While PTG has been viewed as a coping mechanism, it has also been suggested that engaging in cognitive processing of the traumatic event is essential for overcoming it. Either way, this process may help lessen the fear of recurrence.

Several studies have found that people who experience PTG report less fear of recurrence [10]. A survey of 135 female participants with a history of cervical cancer reported higher PTG as a result of self-care self-efficacy. This refers to an individual's belief in their ability to perform the behaviors necessary to manage their health and well-being. This sense of agency helped them feel more resilient in the face of uncertainty.

This may include engaging in physical activity, adopting healthy eating habits, developing effective stress management techniques, and fostering strong interpersonal relationships. Building on the health changes we discussed earlier, this provides further support that changing the trajectory from victim to victor is a decisive step in overcoming the fear of recurrence. The higher the PTG experienced, the less fear of recurrence people report [11].

Success Story

Laurie was diagnosed with breast cancer in her early 60s. Like most people, she was swept into the healthcare system and felt like a faceless number on the never-ending conveyor belt of patients at the hospital. She felt overwhelmed with the information presented to her and struggled to understand the purpose of the medications recommended to her. She was given a long list of potential side effects, with a list of more drugs that would treat those side effects.

Laurie was drawn to holistic medicine and asked about using complementary therapies to support her body during radiation and chemotherapy. However, she felt incredibly dismissed when she asked her doctors questions. She also had many questions about her chemotherapy treatments and questioned whether she needed so many radiation blasts. However, she felt that her questions were met with frustration or indifference and that the healthcare system had a one-size-fits-all approach.

Growing up, Laurie always struggled to find her voice. Throughout her life, she felt like a people pleaser, often saying yes to commitments she didn't want to fulfill. She always found it difficult to speak up for herself and usually found that her own needs and wishes took a distant backseat. But one day, something shifted, and she had a dawning realization that she, and she alone, would have to navigate this. While this felt stressful, it was more of a positive stress, as she thought she would no longer say yes all the time, and she needed to take ownership of her body and her care.

She learned to ask pointed questions to her doctors and nurses and found a doctor who respected her interest in complementary therapies. She managed to prevent many of her side effects with natural therapies and avoided taking so many medications, which was important to her. She also advocated for herself in reducing the number of radiation treatments.

This newfound assertiveness trickled over into other areas of her life, and she no longer extended herself beyond her means. Her cancer diagnosis forced her to confront her insecure nature, and she found what she had always been looking for: her voice. The "good stress" of her cancer journey helped her to value herself more, and while cancer was a painful experience, it ultimately gave her the most valuable lesson of all: how to value herself.

Mindfulness Practice

Imagine a boat gently gliding on the surface of a calm lake. The boat represents your mind, and the water represents your thoughts and emotions. As the boat moves along, it starts to encounter ripples and waves. You notice another boat nearby, driving too quickly and disrupting the stillness. The other boat and the ripples represent distractions and stressors that arise daily. We have two choices. We can focus on the disruption, feeling off-balance, irritated, and annoyed at the other boat for coming so close. Or we can practice mindfulness and lean into the waves, viewing them as calming and gentle, rather than turbulent and disruptive.

This is a metaphor for how mindfulness can help us manage stress. Mindfulness enables you to step back from these stressors, observe them without judgment, and choose how you want to respond to them. Instead of letting stressors consume you, we learn to cultivate a quiet space within ourselves, a space for calm awareness. Studies have found that mindfulness not only reduces fear of recurrence but also improves energy levels [12].

The very essence of mindfulness means bringing compassionate awareness to the present moment. This can help to lessen rumination and worry. Cancer brings about anxieties about the past, present, and future. Cultivating a mindfulness practice redirects drifting, doom-and-gloom thoughts back to the present moment, allowing for distance from repetitive, negative feelings and worries that fuel stress.

Practicing mindfulness through body scans can help you reconnect with your body. You can start to learn the difference between a benign sensation and those that might warrant real medical attention. By easing hypervigilance, mindfulness reduces the mental and physical exhaustion that often accompanies fear of recurrence. Body scans can cultivate an objective understanding of bodily sensations, thereby reducing the mental energy spent on worrying about every ache and pain.

Body Scan Meditation

This practice offers a safe and gentle way to connect with your body's sensations, cultivate awareness of how your body feels on a day-to-day basis, and reduce fear or anxiety about your health.

Begin by finding a comfortable position. You might lie down on your back or sit gently in a chair with your feet flat on the floor. Allow your hands to rest wherever feels natural—perhaps on your lap or by your sides. If it feels right, softly close your eyes.

Let's begin by taking a few slow, intentional breaths. Inhale deeply through your nose, feeling your belly gently rise. And exhale slowly through your mouth, as if sighing out any tension or worry. Take another deep breath in... and out... allowing your body to settle with each breath, inviting a sense of calm to enter your space.

Now, bring your awareness to the top of your head. Notice any sensations there. Perhaps there is a tingling on your scalp or a dull ache. You notice the feeling of your hair. Observe without judgment.

Gently, shift your attention down to your face. Notice your forehead. Is there any tension? See if you can soften it. Relax your eyebrows... your eyelids... your cheeks. Let your jaw hang slightly open, releasing any clenching. Notice your lips... your chin. Allow your whole face to relax.

Now, shift your attention to your neck and shoulders. These are often places where we hold a lot of tension. Without trying to change anything, notice how your neck feels... how your shoulders feel. Are they pulled up toward your ears? Can you invite them to drop gently, allowing them to relax and broaden?

Bring your attention down to your arms, to your elbows, to your forearms, and into your hands. Notice your hands resting wherever they are. Feel the temperature... the texture... the sensations in your fingers, your palms. Are they tense or relaxed? Are they numb or stiff? Let them relax.

Gently guide your awareness into your chest and upper back. Feel the natural rhythm of your breath. Feel your heart beating. Notice any sensations in your rib cage, your collarbones. If you experience feelings of tightness or anxiety in your chest, simply acknowledge them.

Now, move your awareness to your abdomen and lower back. Notice the soft movements of your belly with each breath. Let your stomach relax, not clenched. If you notice any discomfort or sensations, observe them with an open and accepting awareness.

Shift your attention down into your hips and pelvis. Notice where your body makes contact with the chair or the floor. Is there a stretching sensation, or are you loose?

> *Next, move your awareness down your legs, into your thighs and knees. Notice how they feel. Are there aches? Notice the everyday sensations you feel.*
>
> *Then, gently bring your attention down to your calves and shins, and finally, into your feet. Notice your ankles, the tops of your feet, your heels, and your toes. Feel the connection of your feet with the ground beneath you. Notice any tingling, warmth, or coolness. Allow your feet to feel completely relaxed and supported.*
>
> *Now, take a moment to sense your entire body as a whole. From the top of your head to the tips of your toes. Notice your breath flowing through your entire being. Feel the profound stillness and presence that is always available to you, beneath any thoughts or worries.*
>
> *If thoughts of fear, worry about recurrence, or discomfort arise, that is entirely normal. Instead of pushing them away, acknowledge them as they appear, like clouds in the sky. Offer them a gentle "hello," and then gently guide your attention back to the sensation of your breath or to the overall feeling of your body. You are safe. You are present.*
>
> *Rest here for a few more moments, simply being with your body and your breath. You are building resilience simply by noticing.*
>
> *When you're ready to bring this practice to a close gently, begin to deepen your breath once more. Feel the support beneath you. Gently wiggle your fingers and toes, and allow yourself to come back slowly and softly.*

By bringing awareness to the body, we are reminded how it feels daily, and that sometimes unpleasant sensations are normal and common. This differentiates normal bodily sensations from alarming ones, allowing you to feel less hypervigilant and worried about recurrence.

Psychedelic-assisted Therapy for Trauma

Anyone can develop post-traumatic stress (PTS) after a frightening or serious life event. Many cancer survivors experience some degree of PTS, whether from the trauma of treatments or the threat to their life. PTS can manifest through nightmares, flashbacks, persistent intrusive thoughts, avoidance of specific places, hypervigilance, feelings of shame, or difficulty sleeping. People might also feel anxious, depressed, tearful, and angry.

Treatments for PTS typically include antidepressants or antianxiety medications, which often prove ineffective. Psychedelic therapy involves administering hallucinogenic substances, and current research is supporting its effectiveness for severe PTS from life events other than cancer [13]. Hence, the interest has surfaced as to whether psychedelics can lessen the fear of recurrence.

A hallucinogenic state allegedly enables a person to enter an altered level of consciousness, facilitating deeper emotional healing and personal growth. Feedback from studies conducted so far has revealed that after a psychedelic therapy experience, people experience more self-compassion and have lower stress when recalling a stressful event [14]. Studies have also demonstrated that psychedelics decrease emotional intensity, helping people to process traumatic memories [15]. These therapies also enhance mindfulness-related skills and acceptance, all of which help people who have experienced PTS cope with challenging memories [16].

As interest in psychedelic therapy is mounting, governments around the world are getting on board. Australia became the world's first country to legalize the medical use of psychedelics. As psychedelics remain controlled substances in many jurisdictions, access to these medications requires special access programs or enrollment in clinical trials. Trials are currently underway in the United States and Canada.

Some countries, like Canada, allow private clinics to operate and have gained approval to administer specific psychedelic therapies, such as ketamine. However, these services are out-of-pocket expenses and may not be accessible to everyone.

While more research needs to be conducted, at this time, psychedelics have been found to be safe, and patients report emotional breakthroughs. This is something to consider for a severe FCR.

Cognitive Behavioral Therapy

Like many other psychological conditions, talk therapy is also effective in helping to reduce the FCR. Various forms of cognitive behavioral therapy (CBT) have been shown to help, including Managing Cancer and Living Meaningfully Therapy (CALM), Fear of Recurrence Therapy (FORT), and Acceptance and Commitment Therapy (ACT). You can search for a qualified psychologist in your area who can provide support.

Two apps have been found helpful for therapy geared toward fear of recurrence, called iThrive and iConquerFear. App-based technology is convenient and affordable, making access to essential techniques for managing fear of recurrence easier.

Conclusion

It is acknowledged that FCR may persist over time, even years after treatment ends. This fear is recognized as one of the most common unmet needs reported by patients with all types and stages of cancer. As a result, both patients and healthcare providers need to be aware of strategies to address it. FCR is a primary contributor to psychological distress and fatigue [17].

If fear of recurrence is strongly present in your life, following lifestyle guidelines for nutrition and exercise is essential. Additionally, there may be other therapies that can help, such as mindfulness and CBT. Reducing fear of recurrence will improve other aspects of life, including mood, sleep, and energy. Therefore, paying attention to this topic cannot be stressed enough.

References

1 Amani O, Ali Mazaheri M, Moghani MM, et al. Mediating effects of rumination on insomnia in cancer survivors: influences of cancer-related fatigue, fear of recurrence and psychological distress. Cancer Med, 2024; 13(18):e70189.
2 Lebel S, Maheu C, Tomei C, et al. Towards the validation of a new, blended theoretical model of fear of cancer recurrence. Psychooncology, 2018; 27(11):2594–2601.
3 Hyland KA, Jacobs JM, Lennes IT, et al. Are cancer survivors following the National Comprehensive Cancer Network health behavior guidelines? An assessment of patients attending a cancer survivorship clinic. J Psychosoc Oncol, 2018; 36:64–81.
4 Hall DL, Jimenez RB, Perez GK, et al. Fear of cancer recurrence: a model examination of physical symptoms, emotional distress, and health behaviour change. J Oncol Pract, 2019; 15(9):e787–e797.
5 Cannioto RA, Attwood KM, Davis EW. Adherence to cancer prevention lifestyle recommendations before, during and 2 years after treatment for high-risk breast cancer. JAMA Netw Open, 2023; 6(5):e2311673.
6 Rabbani SA, Patni MA, El-Tanani M, et al. Impact of lifestyle modifications on cancer mortality: a systematic review and meta-analysis. Medicina (Kaunas), 2025; 61(2):307.
7 Kang X, Zhang Q, Wang S, et al. Effect of soy isoflavones on breast cancer recurrence and death for patients receiving adjuvant endocrine therapy. CMAJ, 2010; 182(17):1857–1862.
8 Lee S, Ma C, Shi Q, et al. Sleep and cancer recurrence and survival in patients with resected Stage III colon cancer: findings from CALGB/SWOG 80702 (Alliance). Br J Cancer, 2023; 129(2):283–290.
9 Smith BW, Dalen J, Bernard JF, et al. Posttraumatic growth in non-Hispanic White and Hispanic women with cervical cancer. J Psychosoc Oncol, 2008; 26:91–109.
10 Yun SJ, Kim HY. Factors influencing posttraumatic growth of gynecologic oncology patients undergoing chemotherapy. Korean J Women Health Nurs, 2019; 25;409–422.

11 Zhang X, Yuan M, Yue Y, et al. Fear of cancer recurrence and coping strategies among patients with oral cancer: the impact on post-traumatic growth. BMC Psychol, 2025; 13:162.

12 Park S, Sato Y, Takita Y, et al. Mindfulness-based cognitive therapy for psychological distress, fear of cancer recurrence, fatigue, spiritual well-being and quality of life in patients with breast cancer—a randomized controlled trial. J Pain Symptom Manag, 2020; 60(2):381.

13 Mitchell JM, Bogenschutz M, Lilienstein A, et al. MDMA-assisted therapy for severe PTSD: a randomized, double-blind, placebo-controlled Phase 3 study. Nat Med, 2021; 27(6):1025–1033.

14 Kamboj SK, Kilford EJ, Minchin S, et al. Recreational 3,4-methylenedioxy-N-methylamphetamine (MDMA) or 'ecstasy' and self-focused compassion: preliminary steps in the development of a therapeutic psychopharmacology of contemplative practices. J Psychopharmacol, 2015; 29(9):961–970.

15 Mueller F, Lenz C, Dolder PC, et al. Acute effects of LSD on amygdala activity during processing of fearful stimuli in healthy subjects. Translational Psych, 2017; 7(4):e1084.

16 Soler J, Elices M, Franques A, et al. Exploring the therapeutic potential of Ayahuasca: acute intake increases mindfulness-related capacities. Psychopharmacol, 2016; 233(5):823–829.

17 Simard S, Thewes B, Humphris G, et al. Fear of cancer recurrence in adult cancer survivors: a systematic review of quantitative studies. J Cancer Surviv, 2013; 7:300–322.

Part V

Physical Disturbances

14

Restoring Your Sleep Rhythm

The worst thing in the world is to try to sleep, and not to

—F. Scott Fitzgerald

This chapter is for you if:

- You feel as if you've always had trouble sleeping.
- Your sleep has worsened significantly after cancer treatment.
- You struggle to fall asleep or stay asleep.
- You feel like you are not well-rested in the morning and need to nap throughout the day.
- You are using sleep medications and are seeking suggestions to enhance your sleep.

Before we examine how insomnia specifically affects cancer survivors, let's take a moment to acknowledge the importance of sleep. Sleep plays a crucial role in mental restoration, mood, memory, and focus. It bolsters our immune system and helps regulate hormone levels. A good night's sleep benefits our cardiovascular health and supports weight management. Essentially, it acts as a nightly reset button, enabling your body to function at its best. Sleep is governed by an internal "clock" that responds to external cues like light, darkness, and food intake.

Addressing and improving sleep is paramount because over half of cancer survivors experience sleep disturbance, including difficulty falling and staying asleep, excessive daytime sleepiness, circadian rhythm disruptions, and poor sleep quality [1]. When sleep becomes elusive, it touches every part of your well-being.

Sleep disturbance is not only strongly associated with cancer-related fatigue, but it also puts you at a higher risk of obesity, hypertension [2], diabetes [3], cardiovascular disease, and depression. Cancer survivors who do not sleep well

Beyond Cancer Fatigue: A Path to Reclaiming Energy, First Edition. Jessa Landmann, ND.

have an increased risk of a recurrence [4]. This is likely because a lack of sleep is associated with a low immune system and increased inflammation [5]. Frequent nighttime arousals are also associated with a higher risk of mortality in many cancer types, including patients with lung cancer [6] and colon cancer [7].

This is not meant to cause fear or worry. Information is power, and it is vitally important to share information that will directly affect your well-being. This book aims to help you explore and identify factors in your life that impact your energy levels. Improving certain aspects, such as sleep, will have a positive impact on your long-term health.

Factors contributing to sleep disruption include ongoing inflammation from cancer treatments, as well as medication-induced side effects, such as hot flashes or pain. Restless legs is also common [8], as well as disordered breathing, such as sleep apnea [9]. Emotional stress and cortisol also take their toll on sleep, disrupting your circadian rhythm.

But rest assured (pun intended), this chapter offers many strategies and therapeutic options, and hopefully, you will regain the sleep that has eluded you for so long.

REFLECTION POINT
As you work through the rest of the chapter, begin jotting down notes in your journal about anything that resonates with you regarding factors that might be contributing to poor nightly sleep. Then, you can start recording the treatment suggestions you are most interested in trying to help restore your sleep rhythm.

Stress, Cortisol, and Sleep

Your body's stress hormone, cortisol, typically follows a natural rhythm, known as the circadian rhythm. It peaks in the morning to give you the energy to get you going, and then gradually declines throughout the day. Cortisol levels are low in the evening, signaling the body to start slowing down and preparing for sleep. Cortisol should then steadily decrease throughout the night, reaching its lowest point around the middle of the night.

However, when you don't sleep well, this natural rhythm gets thrown off. People who wake up repeatedly during the night or don't get enough total sleep often show higher-than-normal cortisol levels. People with insomnia produce a greater amount of cortisol throughout the day than people without insomnia [10], and this has been found in women with breast and ovarian cancers [11].

When daytime cortisol levels are higher than usual, nighttime cortisol levels are also higher [12]. High daytime cortisol levels can be caused by emotional stress, and as a result, our bodies may struggle to transition into sleep at night.

Even years after treatment, cancer survivors continue to face significant challenges with stress and sleep. It's been found that roughly 33% of breast cancer survivors [13] and prostate cancer survivors [14] struggle with sleep, more than five years out. Poor sleep was directly linked to high rates of stress, high cortisol levels, and depression [15].

Restless Legs

Restless legs syndrome (RLS) is a neurological condition that causes an uncontrollable urge to move the legs. It is often worse at nighttime or during periods of rest, and typically improves with movement. People with RLS may also experience sensations in the legs, such as tingling or itching. As RLS generally occurs at night, people can experience disrupted sleep, fatigue, and daytime sleepiness.

Restless legs is an under-recognized and therefore under-discussed issue that may cause sleep problems in people with cancer. Chemotherapy may increase the risk of RLS, and one study found that about 21% of people undergoing cancer treatment had RLS, more than double the risk of the general population [16]. When people also had depression or anxiety, RLS symptoms were worse. Increased risk of RLS is also seen in survivors of breast cancer being treated with aromatase inhibitors [17].

Additionally, cancer survivors are notoriously iron-deficient, and iron deficiency is recognized to be a contributor to RLS. Approximately 35–50% of people with iron deficiency may experience RLS [18]. Therefore, checking for iron status is an integral part of a sleep assessment.

Sleep Apnea

Here is a bold statement: all cancer survivors who suffer from poor sleep and daytime sleepiness should be screened for sleep apnea. A recent meta-analysis found that 46% of cancer survivors have sleep apnea [19]. Sleep apnea causes periods of non-breathing during sleep, leading to low oxygen levels and, consequently, very low energy levels. Sleep apnea may be a risk factor for the development of cancer [20], as well as cancer recurrence [21]. Sleep apnea is also well recognized to be associated with the development of cardiovascular disease, such as stroke and heart attack. Therefore, there is strong support for screening cancer survivors for sleep apnea.

Certain groups are at a higher risk of developing sleep apnea. People who have been treated for head and neck cancers may have swelling and damage to the throat or nose, and have high rates of sleep apnea [22]. Individuals with a 10% weight gain have a six-fold increased risk of developing sleep apnea [23]. And as discussed in Chapter 6, post-menopausal women have an increased risk of sleep apnea as well.

As we can see, there are a variety of reasons cancer survivors have insomnia or poor sleep quality. A comprehensive sleep assessment would include testing for inflammation, iron status, and cortisol levels, as well as obtaining a referral for a sleep study to rule out sleep apnea.

Integrative Therapies for Insomnia

Cognitive Behavioral Therapy for Insomnia (CBT-I)

CBT-I has demonstrated efficacy in helping cancer patients struggling with insomnia, and is recommended as first-line therapy. CBT-I comprises stimulus control, sleep restriction, relaxation training, sleep hygiene, and cognitive restructuring. A meta-analysis found that CBT-I reduced insomnia severity, shortened the time to fall asleep, and increased the time spent sleeping, with these effects lasting up to 6 months [24].

CBT-I can be delivered in person, but it can also be effective when delivered via telehealth for those living in remote areas. Self-help therapy is an effective way to embark on CBT-I, such as the Sleep Reset program co-created by scientists at Yale and Stanford. You may also prefer an app-based program—iCANSleep is Canada's first clinically validated app for helping cancer survivors get a good night's sleep.

While this book cannot replace a trained therapist, let's discuss some CBT-I concepts you can start putting into practice tonight.

Stimulus Control

Stimulus control is designed to help people reconnect with their bedtime routine [25]. Interventions aim to make bedtime a positive experience and to diminish behaviors that may be hindering sleep. Creating a better bedroom environment, associating the bed with sleep, avoiding sleeping elsewhere, and reconditioning the body to fall asleep all fall under the umbrella of stimulus control.

Techniques used in stimulus control are as follows:

Technique	Description
"The bed is for sleep and sex only. No other activities should occur in the bed."	This works to re-establish the bed as a place of sleep and sex, and nothing else.
"Avoid daytime napping."	Daytime napping can reduce the drive for sleep at nighttime. During the day, sleep debt is built; without enough sleep debt sleeping at night can be difficult.
"Eliminate visual and auditory distractions at night."	Sleeping in a dark, quiet, cool room makes it easier to fall asleep. Eliminating distractions from gadgets and light will help with sleep.
"Create a bedtime ritual that allows relaxation to start before bedtime."	Rituals can include warm herbal teas, soft music, a warm bath, journaling, and meditation.
"Go to bed and wake up at the same time each day."	Setting a strict schedule will condition the body to know when to expect sleep and when to expect arousal. Even on weekends, go to bed at the same time and wake up at the same time.
"Do not spend more than 20 minutes awake in bed."	If not asleep after 20 minutes, get out of bed and engage in a neutral activity. If getting up, avoid television, screens, or eating. Return to bed when sleepy again.

Success Story

Janet was diagnosed with metastatic breast cancer, and she came to see me primarily for low energy levels. She reported that she could barely make it through the day for more than two hours at a time without needing to nap. This didn't affect her ability to sleep at night, as she would often nap throughout the day and sleep nine to 10 hours at night. Janet also struggled with depression, which could have been a factor in the desire to sleep a lot.

Her physical activity level was low, as even walking around the block left her feeling fatigued. This was likely also contributing to her fatigue, as we know that low physical activity and sedentary behavior sap our energy levels.

Sleeping too much in a 24-hour period paradoxically results in lower energy levels. Therefore, I advised her to avoid taking a nap during the day, even though it would be challenging for her. During the time she would usually nap, she would

(Continued)

(Continued)

work on art projects with her grandchildren, talk to a friend, or do something that helped her connect with a loved one.

After two weeks without daytime naps, she noticed her energy levels improved and she was able to go for longer walks. Previously, she could only walk about 10 minutes, but now she walks about 45 minutes per day, and has found a friend to do this with.

By replacing naps with meaningful and joyful activities, she improved her mood, her sense of social connection, and, of course, her energy. All of this was possible by simply eliminating daytime naps.

Sleep Restriction

Sleep restriction is a technique designed to strengthen the connection between your bed and actual sleep. The idea is simple: if you spend too much time lying awake in bed, your brain starts to associate the bed with wakefulness and frustration, rather than rest.

By restricting the amount of time you spend in bed only when you're actually sleeping, you essentially "re-train" your brain to associate the bed with sleep. The ultimate goal is to increase your sleep efficiency—meaning that the vast majority of time you spend in bed is spent soundly asleep, not tossing and turning.

Sleep efficiency can be calculated as follows:

$$\text{Total sleep time/Total time in bed} \times 100 = \%\text{efficiency}.$$

For example, if someone goes to bed at 11 pm and gets up at 7 am, they would have spent a total of eight hours in bed. However, if that person did not fall asleep until 1 am, then the total sleep time is only six hours. Sleep efficiency would be calculated as:

$$\text{6 hours total sleep time/8 hours total time in bed} \times 100 = 75\%.$$

While there is some variability in what the desired sleep efficiency should be, most of the literature generally agrees that the goal is between 80 and 90%. The steps for restriction are as follows:

Step 1: Keep a sleep diary for one to two weeks to monitor your sleep, then calculate sleep efficiency as described above.

Step 2: Adjust the total time in bed to match the total sleep time, while keeping the wake-up time constant. For example, if you don't fall asleep until 1 am, then go to bed at that time.

This often means individuals go to bed later, which can be difficult. However, over time, your body should become accustomed to falling asleep when you go to bed, and you can eventually return to an earlier bedtime.

Step 3: Continue calculating sleep efficiency until you reach a desired range of 80–90%.

Relaxation Training

Getting the body into a relaxed state is essential to prepare the mind to sleep. Relaxation techniques activate the parasympathetic nervous system, which prepares the brain and body for a restful night's sleep. Relaxation techniques are effective for sleep because they can lower cortisol, lower heart rate and lower feelings of anxiety or depression. Relaxation techniques include guided imagery and diaphragmatic breathing.

Guided imagery uses the power of our imagination to produce a positive mind–body experience. You can be your own creative guide, and while lying in bed, imagine yourself anywhere you find beautiful and that you associate with relaxation. Maybe that's sitting on top of a mountain by yourself, or maybe your mind has you lying on the grass under the night sky, stargazing.

The reason guided imagery is such a powerful tool is that neuroscience has shown that our brains cannot distinguish between real and imagined situations. Just think of it—have you ever imagined something frightening happening to you or a loved one? How has that affected your body? Did you experience stomach pain or feel your heart rate increase? What we imagine can feel very real.

Therefore, imagining yourself in a relaxing environment can trick your brain into thinking you are there, helping you achieve better sleep.

Diaphragmatic breathing is a relaxation technique we have yet to discuss in this book. Breathing techniques can be used for stress management and to alleviate sleep difficulties. We discussed box breathing in Chapter 12. Slow, deep breathing activates the parasympathetic nervous system, which induces sleepiness and deep relaxation. Just 20 minutes of diaphragmatic breathing, performed twice daily, can lower cortisol levels, anxiety, blood pressure, and heart rate, and improve sleep and energy levels [26].

Script for Diaphragmatic Breathing Exercise

As you lie in bed, allow yourself to get as comfortable as possible. Feel the support of your mattress beneath you. Let your body grow heavy, soft, and still.

Gently bring your awareness to your breath. Notice the natural rise and fall of your chest and belly. Now, place one hand gently on your chest and the other hand on your belly, just below your rib cage. This will help you feel the movement of your breath.

The goal here is to breathe deeply into your belly, not just your chest. Imagine your belly is a balloon that you gently inflate with each inhale and slowly deflate with each exhale.

Let's begin. Take a slow, gentle breath in through your nose, feeling your belly hand rise, pushing your hand upwards. Try to keep your chest hand as still as possible.

Now, slowly exhale through your mouth, letting your belly fall gently downwards, releasing all the air.

Let's do that again. Inhale slowly through your nose, feeling your belly expand...and exhale slowly through your mouth, letting your belly soften and fall. Continue this gentle rhythm. Inhale deeply, feeling your belly rise and fall.

Notice how your body begins to relax with each inhale and exhale. As your belly gently rises and falls, imagine that you are releasing any tension from your mind, from your shoulders, from your entire body.

This deep, calming breath sends a signal to your body that it's safe to rest and let go. It helps to quiet your nervous system, allowing you to transition smoothly from wakefulness into sleep.

Allow yourself to fully sink into the comfort of your bed, supported by this gentle, deep breath. Each inhale brings calm; each exhale guides you deeper into relaxation.

You are safe. You are at peace. And you are ready for a truly restful, restorative sleep. Continue to breathe in this gentle rhythm as you drift off into a deep, restful sleep.

Exercise

When it comes to exercise and sleep, researchers have explored a range of activities, from running and weightlifting to yoga, Tai chi, and even walking, and have found benefits across the board. Consistent with the message of other chapters in this book, you should always aim for a moderate- to vigorous-intensity workout (when you're breathing hard), where you are using your large muscle groups (like your legs), at least three to five times per week.

Most studies find that exercise results in longer sleep times, which in turn translates to better energy levels during the day [27]. Exercise decreases cortisol levels, which is likely one of the main ways exercise improves sleep. This makes it an incredibly valuable tool worth exploring for anyone seeking to enhance their energy levels and overall well-being.

There has been much debate about the optimal timing of exercise. Some claim that evening exercise is too invigorating and leads to increased nighttime arousal, which can interfere with sleep. Studies have yielded mixed results, with some indicating that both evening and morning exercise are equally effective in improving sleep [28].

What matters most is finding what works for you—exercise at the time of day when you feel most energetic and it fits your routine best.

Acupuncture

Acupuncture is as effective [29], or even more effective [30], than commonly used prescription sleep medications. Acupuncture was also found to be almost as effective as CBT-I in cancer survivors [31]. Acupuncture can improve sleep in people who have chronic pain [32] and in women who are experiencing psychological distress, such as depression and anxiety [33]. Acupuncture can help individuals fall asleep more quickly, prolong the duration of sleep, and reduce daytime sleepiness [34]. Therefore, acupuncture is strongly supported as a beneficial treatment for sleep difficulties.

CLINICAL PEARL

My acupuncture protocol for treating sleep issues includes the following points: LV3, SP6, ST36, LV8, HT7, PC6, GV20, Anmian, Shenmen, and Yintang. Acupuncture should ideally be performed twice a week for six weeks, but once a week can also be beneficial.

Treatments for Restless Legs Syndrome (RLS)

Iron Supplementation

Iron deficiency is one of the most recognized causes of RLS, and therefore, it follows that iron supplementation should be beneficial. Both intravenous and oral iron supplements are effective in reducing leg restlessness, improving sleep quality, and increasing energy levels [35, 36].

CLINICAL PEARL

Iron comes in many forms, and I recommend iron bisglycinate. Take 10–20 mg for six months, along with vitamin C, to help improve iron absorption. If you can get a referral to an iron infusion clinic, two treatments are recommended, spaced one week apart.

Magnesium

Magnesium is commonly taken to relieve muscle cramps and to help with sleep. Therefore, it makes biological sense to add magnesium for RLS. Magnesium is a mild muscle relaxant, and it is very calming to the nervous system. Research confirms that magnesium can be effective for RLS [37].

CLINICAL PEARL

Both magnesium citrate and magnesium oxide can help alleviate RLS symptoms. Start with a dose of 250 mg about 30 minutes before bedtime, and increase to 450 mg as needed until you find relief.

Complementary Treatments for Sleep Apnea

Mediterranean Diet Plus CPAP

If you have been diagnosed with sleep apnea, there is a fascinating study you must know about. While a CPAP machine is the gold standard for treating sleep apnea, nutritional interventions can also be beneficial.

In the study, participants with sleep apnea were divided into two groups: one used only a CPAP machine, while the other combined CPAP therapy with a Mediterranean diet [38]. The results were striking—breathing interruptions improved fivefold in the group following the Mediterranean diet. As a result, these participants slept better and felt more energized during the day.

The Mediterranean diet is naturally anti-inflammatory, and reducing inflammation can help ease sleep apnea symptoms. As discussed in the weight loss chapter, this diet also promotes healthy weight loss, which further benefits people with sleep apnea.

Melatonin

Research supports the safety of long-term use of melatonin for cancer survivors. Melatonin provides longer sleep duration, reduced use of prescription sleep medication [39], decreased cancer fatigue, and improved quality of life [40].

CLINICAL PEARL

If you are new to taking melatonin, start with 1.5 mg 30 minutes before bed. Try this for a few nights and gradually increase your dose to 10 mg until you notice improvements in sleep.

Herbal Therapy for Sleep

Herbs are among the most effective ways to support sleep, particularly for individuals under high stress. Many herbs stimulate the brain centers that promote relaxation and have been found to lower cortisol levels. Due to their long use in traditional medicine, herbal therapies are generally considered safe and can be used by people of all ages.

There are numerous to choose from, and here are some of the most popular, with research to back them up!

Passionflower

Passionflower has been studied in people with insomnia and found to increase total sleep time. Not only did people experience longer sleep, but they also had fewer nighttime awakenings, less stress, better energy, and better ability to function and concentrate at work [41].

CLINICAL PEARL

A passionflower tablet of 600 mg is safe and effective; however, teas can also work well. Take passionflower one hour before bed.

Lemon Balm

Lemon balm is an ancient herb that has been used for over 2,000 years. Lemon balm has been found to improve insomnia, lessen anxiety and depression, lessen stress, and improve concentration [42].

CLINICAL PEARL

Lemon balm, taken in doses of 240–1,000 mg, is safe and effective for improving sleep. Begin with a low dose and gradually increase until you notice an improvement in your sleep.

Valerian

Valerian is another ancient herb that has traditionally been used for nervous disorders, such as anxiety and stress. Like passionflower and lemon balm, it activates centers in the brain that induce drowsiness and relaxation. Valerian helps you to fall asleep, stay asleep, and increase energy [43].

CLINICAL PEARL

Doses range from 300 mg to 600 mg, taken one hour before bed. Valerian can also be consumed as a tea if you prefer.

Light Therapy

Light is one of the main stimuli that signals the body to wake up in the morning and go to sleep at night. Light is one of the main drivers of a regular and happy circadian rhythm, which, as you know by now, can get out of sync after cancer treatments. Exposure to bright white light in the morning helps restore the circadian rhythm and can improve sleep quality not only in cancer survivors [44] but also in those still undergoing chemotherapy [45].

Sleep aside, light therapy is effective for cancer-related fatigue, so even if you don't notice the benefits for your sleep, you may see a boost in energy [46]. One study exposed people to a light box for 30 minutes every morning, within 30 minutes of waking, for four weeks. After this period, the participants reported that their fatigue had disappeared [47].

Light interventions can be both natural and artificial. Artificial sources of light come in the form of light boxes, where people can look into the box for up to 30 minutes at a time. LiteBook is one product that has been used in studies. There are also light glasses, where a source of light is emitted from the lenses, such as Re-Timer glasses.

Seeking out natural sources of light is most recommended, such as a walk outside in the morning light within an hour of waking. Walking outside in natural light offers a wealth of benefits that can't be replicated by staying indoors under artificial lighting. We know that exposure to natural light can boost serotonin levels and reduce stress, anxiety, and depression. By choosing to walk outside, we tap into the restorative power of nature, promoting both physical and mental well-being in a way that artificial light cannot match.

Conclusion

Each person's sleep journey is unique. What works for one person may not work for another. What's important is to start with some basics and go from there. Ensure your room is dark and cool. Establish a bedtime routine, and try one of the herbal teas. Check in with yourself about how stressed you feel going to bed—try a guided imagery or deep breathing exercise. Also, ensure that you rule out potentially serious causes of poor sleep, such as sleep apnea. Creating the conditions for optimal sleep is an ongoing process, and the goal of this chapter was to help promote a sense of peace, tranquility, and a sense of control.

References

1 Al Maqbali M, Al Sinani M, Alsayed A, et al. Prevalence of sleep disturbance in patients with cancer: a systematic review and meta-analysis. Clin Nurs Res, 2022; 31(6):1107–1123.

2 Vgontzas AN, Liao D, Bixler EO, et al. Insomnia with objective short sleep duration is associated with a high risk for hypertension. Sleep, 2009; 32:491–497.

3 Vgontzas AN, Liao D, Pejovic S, et al. Insomnia with objective short sleep duration is associated with type 2 diabetes: a population-based study. Diabetes Care, 2009; 32:1980–1985.

4 Irwin MR. Depression and insomnia in cancer: prevalence, risk factors, and effects on cancer outcomes. Curr Psychiatry Rep, 2013; 15(11):404.

5 Besedovsky L, Lange T, Haack M. The sleep-immune crosstalk in health and disease. Physiol Rev, 2019; 99(3):1325–1380.

6 Gottfried T, Kamer I, Salant I, et al. Self reported sleep quality as prognostic for survival in lung cancer patients. Cancer Manag Res, 2020; 12:313–321.

7 Innominato PF, Spiegel D, Ulusakarya A, et al. Subjective sleep and overall survival in chemotherapy naive patients with metastatic colorectal cancer. Sleep Med, 2015; 16(3):391–398.

8 Davidon JR, Maclean AW, Brundage MD, et al. Sleep disturbance in cancer patients. Soc Sci Med, 2002; 54(9):1309–1321.

9 Friedman M, Landsberg R, Pryor S, et al. The occurrence of sleep-disordered breathing among patients with head and neck cancer, Laryngoscope, 2001; 111(11):1917–1919.

10 Vgontzas AN, Bixler EO, Lin HM, et al. Chronic insomnia is associated with nocturnal activation of the hypothalamic-pituitary-adrenal axis: clinical implications. J Clin Endocrinol Metab. 2001; 86:3787–3794.

11 Lutgendorg SK, Weinrib AZ, Penedo F, et al. Interleukin-6, cortisol and depressive symptoms in ovarian cancer patients. J Clin Oncol, 2008; 26(29):4820–4827.

12 Sephton S, Spiegel D. Circadian disruption in cancer: a neuroendocrine-immune pathway from stress to disease? Brain Behav Immun, 2003; 17(5):321–328.

13 Haque R, Hsu JW, Avila C, et al. Insomnia and susceptibility to depressive symptoms and fatigue in diverse breast cancer survivors. J Womens Health, 2021; 30(11):1604–1615.

14 Herouet S, Savard J, Simard J. Psychological functioning associated with prostate cancer: cross sectional comparison of patients treated with radiotherapy, brachytherapy or surgery. J Pain Symptom Manage, 2005; 30:474–484.

15 Hoyt MA, Bower JE, Irwin MR, et al. Sleep quality and depressive symptoms after prostate cancer: the mechanistic role of cortisol. Behav Neurosci, 2016; 130(3):351–356.

16 Saini A, Berruti A, Ferini-Strambli L, et al. Restless legs syndrome as a cause of sleep disturbances in cancer patients receiving chemotherapy. J Pain Symptom Manag, 2013; 46(1):56–64.

17 Pedersini R, di Mauro P, Amoroso V, et al. Sleep disturbances and restless legs syndrome in postmenopausal women with early breast cancer given adjuvant aromatase inhibitor therapy. Breast, 2022; 66:162–168.

18 Allen RP, Auerbach S, Bahrain H, et al. The prevalence and impact of restless legs syndrome on patients with iron deficiency anemia. Am J Hematol, 2013; 88:261–264.

19 Cao Y, Ning P, Li Q, et al. Cancer and obstructive sleep apnea: an updated meta-analysis. Medicine (Baltimore), 2022; 101(10):e28930.

20 Silly A, Watson NF, Schwartz SM, et al. Sleep apnea and subsequent cancer incidence. Cancer Causes Control, 2019; 29(10):987–994.

21 Rodriguez FF, Lim K, Piker T, et al. Cancer reoccurrence is accelerated by episodic hypoxemia. Sleep, 2024; 47(1):201–202.

22 Huyett P, Kim S, Johnson JT, et al. Obstructive sleep apnea in the irradiated head and neck cancer patient. Laryngoscope, 2017; 127:2673–2677.

23 Peppard PE, Young T, Palta M, et al. Longitudinal study of moderate weight change and sleep-disordered breathing. JAMA, 2000; 284:3015–3021.

24 Johnson JA, Rash JA, Campbell TS, et al. A systematic review and meta-analysis of randomized controlled trials of cognitive behavior therapy for insomnia in cancer survivors. Sleep Med Rev, 2016; 27:20–28.

25 Melton L. Cognitive behavioural therapy for sleep in cancer patients: research, techniques and individual considerations. J Adv Pract Oncol, 2018; 9(7):732–740.

26 Ismail AMA, El Gressy NSSA, Hegazy MD, et al. Effects of diaphragmatic breathing exercise on sleeping quality, cortisol, cardiovascular autonomic functions, depression, and fatigue: a randomized-controlled trial in women with systemic sclerosis. Reumatologia, 2025; 63(2):89–96.

27 Chen R, Wang S, Hu Q, et al. Exercise intervention in middle-aged and elderly individuals with insomnia improves sleep and restores connectivity in the motor network. Transl Psychiatry, 2024; 14(1):159.

28 Shen B, Zheng H, Liu H, et al Differential benefits of 12-week morning vs. evening aerobic exercise on sleep and cardiometabolic health: a randomized controlled trial. Sci Rep, 2025; 15(1):18298.

29 Tu J, Chung WC, Yang CY, et al. Comparison between acupuncture versus zolpidem for the treatment of primary insomnia. Asian J Psychiatr, 2012; 5(3):231–235.

30 Garland SN, Xie SX, Li Q, et al. Comparative effectiveness of electro-acupuncture versus gabapentin for sleep disturbances in breast cancer survivors with hot flashes: a randomized trial. Menopause, 2017; 24(5):517–523.

31 Garland SN, Xie SX, DuHamel K, et al. Acupuncture versus cognitive behavioural therapy for insomnia in cancer survivors: a randomized clinical trial. J Natl Cancer Inst, 2019; 111(12):1323–1331.

32 Yang M, Baser RE, Liou KT, et al. Effect of acupuncture versus usual care on sleep quality in cancer survivors with chronic pain: a secondary analysis of a randomized clinical trial. Cancer, 2023; 129(13):2084–2094.

33 Mao J, Farrar JT, Bruner D, et al. Electroacupuncture for fatigue, sleep and psychological distress in breast cancer patients with aromatase inhibitor-related arthralgia: a randomized trial. Cancer, 2014; 120(23):3744–3751.

34 Wang WJ, Zhao N, Yu XT, et al. Bushen aashen acupuncture for perimenopausal insomnia of kidney-yin deficiency: a randomized controlled trial. Zhongguo Zhen Jiu, 2023; 43(6):634–638.

35 Macher S, Herster C, Holter M, et al. The effect of parenteral or oral iron supplementation on fatigue, sleep, quality of life and restless legs syndrome in iron deficiency blood donors: a secondary analysis of the IronWoMan RCT. Nutrients, 2020; 12:1313.

36 Short V, Allen R, Earley CJ, et al. A randomized double-blind pilot study to evaluate the efficacy, safety and tolerability of intravenous iron versus oral iron for the treatment of restless legs syndrome in patients with iron deficiency anemia. Am J Hematol, 2024; 99(6):1077–1083.

37 Gorantla S, Ravisankar A, Trotti LM. Magnesium citrate monotherapy improves restless legs syndrome symptoms and multiple suggested immobilization test scores in an open-label pilot study. J Clin Sleep Med, 2024; 20(8):1357–1361.

38 Georgoulis M, Yiannakouris N, Kechribari I, et al. Dose-response relationship between weight loss and improvements in obstructive sleep apnea severity after a diet/lifestyle intervention: secondary analysis of the "MIMOSA" randomized clinical trial. J Clin Sleep Med, 2022; 18(5):1251–1261.

39 Vaziri N, Shakourifar M, Sattari P, et al. Melatonin aids in treating mood and sleep problems resulting from hormonal therapy in breast cancer patients: a randomized, double-blinded, placebo controlled trial. Iran J Pharm Res, 2025; 23(1):e156581.

40 Javadinia SA, Amlashi ZK, Pashaki AS. Long-term melatonin administration and cancer fatigue in breast cancer patients: a randomized controlled trial. ESMO Open, 2023; 8(1):101357.

41 Harit MK, Mundhe N, Tamoli Sr S, et al. Randomized, double-blind, placebo-controlled, clinical study of Passiflora incarnata in participants with stress and sleep problems. Cureus, 2024; 16(3):e56530.

42 Matthews IM, Eastwood J, Lamport DJ, et al. Clinical efficacy and tolerability of lemon balm (Melissa officinalis) in psychological well-being. Nutrients, 2020; 16(20):3545.

43 Fernández-San-Martín MI, Masa-Font R, Palacios-Soler L. Effectiveness of valerian on insomnia: a meta-analysis of randomized placebo-controlled trials. Sleep Med, 2010; 11:505–511.

44 Fox RS, Baik SH, McGinty H, et al. Feasibility and preliminary efficacy of a bright light intervention in ovarian and endometrial cancer survivors. Int J Behav Med, 2021; 28(1):83–95.

45 Wu HS, Davis JE, Chen L. Bright light shows promise in improving sleep, depression, and quality of life in women with breast cancer during chemotherapy: findings of a pilot study. Chronobiol Int, 2021; 38(5):694–704.

46 Johnson JA, Garland SN, Carlson LE. Bright light therapy improves cancer-related fatigue in cancer survivors: a randomized controlled trial. J Cancer Surviv, 2018; 12(2):206–215.

47 Redd WH, Valdimarsdottir H, Wu LM, et al. Systematic light exposure in the treatment of cancer-related fatigue: a preliminary study. Psychooncology, 2014; 23(12):1431–1434.

15

Quieting Pain to Recharge

As long as you are breathing, there is more right with you than there is wrong, no matter how ill or hopeless you may feel

—Jon Kabat-Zinn

This chapter is for you if:

- You have developed chronic pain since undergoing cancer treatment.
- You had pain before cancer treatment, but it has worsened.
- You take pain medication and wonder what other therapies could help you.

Being a cancer survivor should make you feel like nothing can bring you down, yet for many, they are left with two challenges that undermine that triumph: pain and fatigue. These are not merely two separate symptoms, but aspects of the cancer journey that are deeply intertwined. Understanding this crucial link is one of the first steps toward feeling better. This chapter explores effective strategies to overcome the grip of pain and lead a more active and vibrant life.

Pain impacts individuals throughout their cancer journey. It's estimated that 40–60% of cancer survivors will continue to experience pain after their treatment ends [1]. This can be a debilitating symptom that profoundly affects every aspect of a person's life. It can diminish hope, making it difficult to truly move forward and focus on what matters.

Fatigue and pain are closely connected. Usually, the more intense the pain, the lower a person's energy levels. Pain can lead to fatigue because it interrupts sleep, and the sheer mental effort required to endure it can be exhausting. Conversely, fatigue can amplify the perception of pain, eroding your ability to cope. This creates a vicious cycle that can make someone feel like they are in a downward spiral.

Beyond Cancer Fatigue: A Path to Reclaiming Energy, First Edition. Jessa Landmann, ND.

There are many reasons for long-standing pain. First, chronic post-surgical pain is common. It is estimated that 35% of women who have had surgery for breast cancer will continue to experience pain [2]. All surgeries can create unwanted side effects from scar tissue buildup, pain near the incision, and nerve pain.

Second, neuropathic pain is caused by some classes of chemotherapy. It is estimated that one in three cancer survivors with pain is struggling with neuropathy [3]. This can leave people with discomfort, numbness, and tingling in their hands and feet, and unfortunately, even the best pain medications have limited success.

A third type of pain is joint and muscle discomfort. Breast cancer survivors who need to take anti-hormone medications often report joint and muscle pain, which is a significant reason why women stop these treatments. Many individuals who have undergone chemotherapy also report experiencing general "aches and pains."

A fourth type of pain, often overlooked and underestimated, is digestive pain. Frequently referred to as "chemo belly," it can manifest as bloating, gas, cramping, constipation, diarrhea, and general digestive discomfort. This is common among people who have undergone chemotherapy or radiation therapy to the abdomen or pelvis.

Addressing cancer pain isn't just about managing a symptom; it's about maintaining dignity, restoring quality of life, and empowering individuals to live as fully as possible. When pain is widespread, it can become the primary focus, overshadowing moments of joy and connection. By actively and compassionately managing pain, we can help break this cycle, fostering a sense of vitality and enabling individuals to reclaim precious energy for healing, connection, and living life on their own terms.

This chapter explores how complementary therapies can help reduce pain, improve sleep, boost mood, and increase energy, ultimately enabling you to return to what you love doing.

Complementary Therapies for Pain Management

Holistic therapies are not always about choosing one path over another. Often, the beauty lies in strategically combining the best of both worlds. The coordinated use of evidence-based complementary therapies alongside conventional treatments frequently yields superior results.

Complementary therapies aren't meant to replace your prescription pain medications, but to amplify their effectiveness, especially when pain is severe. The goal is to work in harmony. Holistic therapies can reduce the necessary doses of pain medication, significantly cutting down on unwanted side effects. The ultimate aim is a collaborative effort in which conventional and complementary medicines unite to achieve superior pain management and a higher quality of life.

Acupuncture

In the area of pain management, acupuncture is truly the top choice. There is solid evidence that acupuncture helps with all four types of pain mentioned: post-surgical pain, neuropathic pain, joint and muscle pain, and digestive pain.

Post-surgical Pain

Managing post-surgical pain is essential because it can influence recovery, mobility, and long-term health. After surgery, early movement is crucial, as it helps prevent serious complications such as blood clots. Moving around early begins the process of rebuilding strength and function. Therefore, if pain is significant after surgery, mobilization may need to be postponed.

One of the strongest arguments for effective post-surgical pain management is that unmanaged acute pain following surgery often predicts the development of chronic pain later on, sometimes even years afterward [4].

Several studies have shown that acupuncture after surgery can reduce pain and may also accelerate the recovery of affected organs to their normal functioning [5]. Acupuncture is effective for post-surgical pain after a prostatectomy, and may be as effective, or more so, than prescription pain medication [6].

Acupuncture also offers powerful support prior to surgery. Consider asking your acupuncturist about specialized press tacks applied to acupoints LI4, PC6, and SP6 before your procedure. These tiny, comfortable needles stay in place until they naturally fall off, without increasing the risk of infection, causing bleeding, or interfering with surgery. Research confirms that applying these tacks preoperatively can significantly decrease both pain and vomiting afterward [7].

Success Story
Alma came to my office six months after her double mastectomy for breast cancer. She chose not to have reconstruction and was left with two very painful incisions on her chest. She felt a burning sensation around the surgical sites, and the

(Continued)

(Continued)

skin was extremely tender to touch. She always wore loose tops when out, and she mentioned that at home, she often went topless to avoid clothing touching her skin.

She rated the pain as a 7 out of 10, and it significantly disrupted her sleep and quality of life. She had tried a few over-the-counter pain medications, but to no avail. She felt like she was mentally recovering from the trauma of her surgery, but the pain was a daily reminder of what she had experienced.

I recommended acupuncture to relieve the pain. For this type of discomfort, needles were placed parallel to the ribs above and below the incisions, and points like Shenmen, ST36, LI4, and LV3 were also used.

After six treatments, Alma reported that her pain was entirely gone. She was sleeping through the night and experienced less distress during the day. She was completely surprised, as was I, given the intensity of the pain, and felt like she was regaining her life.

Neuropathic Pain

Peripheral neuropathy is nerve damage that can occur from some types of chemotherapy. It usually appears in the hands and feet and can be problematic, as it may cause tingling, shooting sensations, numbness, increased sensitivity to touch, or burning pain. For those affected, it can significantly impact quality of life, leaving individuals feeling helpless.

While sensory changes are most commonly linked to neuropathic pain, muscle cramps are also an under-recognized symptom of neuropathy. In one study, among people who experienced neuropathy following a stem-cell transplant, 50% reported muscle cramps in the lower limbs, often described as debilitating [8]. Some individuals experience muscle cramps several times per week, usually at inconvenient times, such as while driving or in the middle of the night.

Acupuncture has been shown to help with sensory changes and cramps. A recent meta-analysis that reviewed 11 different studies involving 740 people concluded that acupuncture has strong potential for relieving pain, restoring sensation, and improving quality of life [9].

CLINICAL PEARL

I have had great success with the following protocol for neuropathy in the feet. If you see an acupuncturist, show them this section. "Insert needles bilaterally at ST36, SP9, SP6, and LV3. With an electrical stimulation unit, attach leads from ST36 to LV3, and a separate lead attaching SP9 and SP6. Set the frequency to 2–10 Hz for 25–30 minutes. Treatment frequency is best done twice per week for six to eight weeks."

If there is no improvement after four sessions, add Bafeng and KD3.

Success Story

Dennis came to see me two years after he had been diagnosed with kidney cancer. He was on a medication that caused severe muscle cramps in his feet. He described them as causing his toes to splay out, and become rigid and unmovable, with a pain intensity of an 8 out of 10. He was recently involved in a motor vehicle accident, as he had a painful foot cramp while driving and was unable to apply the brakes.

I performed the above acupuncture protocol for four sessions, and he reported that his muscle cramps were resolved. I continued to see Dennis as a patient for many years, never for the cramps to return.

Joint and Muscle Pain

A common cause of joint pain is from aromatase inhibitors, such as Letrozole or Anastrozole, prescribed for the treatment of breast cancer. This musculoskeletal side effect is one of the most prevalent with these drugs, and in some cases, the pain's severity leads patients to discontinue therapy.

Acupuncture is one of the top treatments endorsed for the treatment of this type of pain [10]. If you can't go to an acupuncturist, acupressure has also been shown to be effective. Acupressure involves applying pressure to acupuncture points for three minutes at a time, once or twice per day. Studies have shown that this is an effective home-based treatment that women can do themselves [11].

CLINICAL PEARL

Press on each of the points below for three minutes at a time, consecutively. You can do this as many times as you wish in a day, even just once. If you prefer to see an acupuncturist, you can show them these points as my recommended pain protocol.

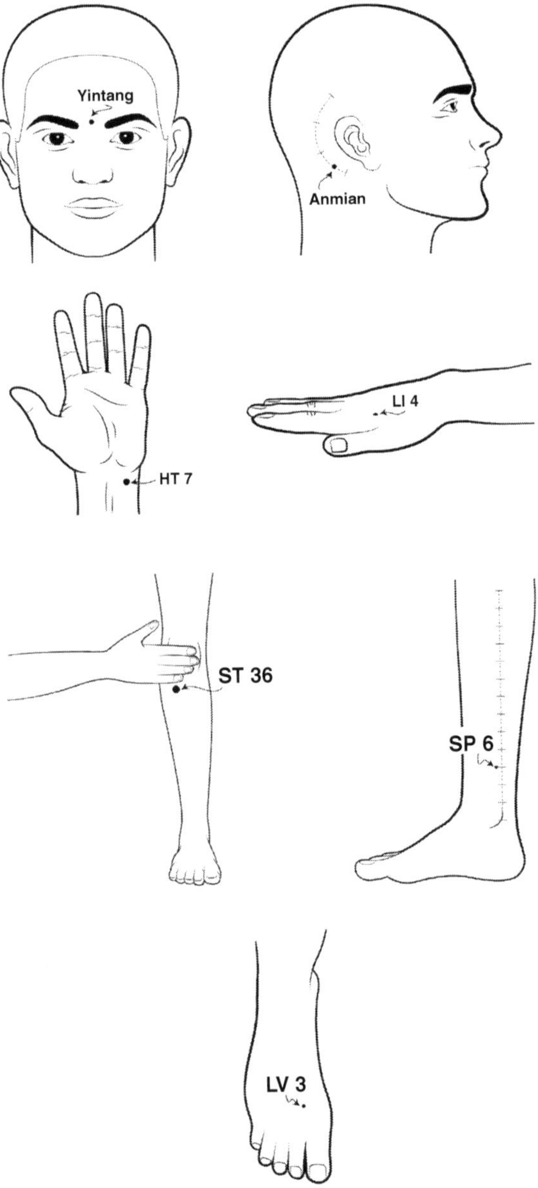
Yintang
Anmian
HT 7
LI 4
ST 36
SP 6
LV 3

Digestive Pains

As described earlier, bloating, constipation, diarrhea, and generalized abdominal discomfort are common in cancer survivors, forming part of the picture known as "chemo belly." Acupuncture is highly effective in relieving all of these discomforts, often with long-lasting impact [12].

However, if someone complains of chemo belly, it is vital to rule out a condition called small intestinal bacterial overgrowth (SIBO). SIBO is an abnormal overgrowth of bacteria in the small intestine, where bacteria don't normally reside. Symptoms of SIBO are constipation or diarrhea, bloating, skin issues, and fatigue. It has been estimated that about 65% of patients with colon, stomach and pancreatic cancers have SIBO [13].

CLINICAL PEARL

If you have ongoing digestive pains, consider asking for a SIBO breath test. If detected, it can be treated with either antibiotics or herbal therapy, both of which are equally effective. A comprehensive SIBO protocol is too detailed to include here, however, please consult an integrative practitioner who can assist you with testing and treatment.

Exercise

Though it may feel counterintuitive, movement is one of the body's most powerful tools for reducing pain. The saying "motion is lotion" holds true: movement lubricates joints, boosts blood flow to muscles, and enhances the delivery of vital nutrients and oxygen to your tissues.

Exercise also releases natural painkillers, called endorphins. These bind to receptors in the brain, lowering our perception of pain. Exercise is known to reduce inflammation, which is another way it helps alleviate pain. Exercise naturally lifts your mood, as explained in Chapter 11. The mental benefits of exercise are clear, and when our mood improves, pain levels tend to decrease.

Exercise is an effective way to manage generalized aches and pains, as well as joint pains associated with hormone-blocking agents [14]. High-intensity interval training (HIIT) is an effective strategy for pain relief and can be conveniently done anywhere [15].

CLINICAL PEARL

An effective HIIT workout you can do anywhere: 30 squats, 20 speed skaters, 20 push-ups, 20 bicycle crunches, 50 jumping jacks, 20 high knees, and 20 glute bridges. Take 30-second breaks in between each exercise. Repeat twice.

Music Therapy

Music therapy is an excellent complementary treatment for many reasons. First, it considers personal preference—if you enjoy classical music, listen to it. If you prefer opera or jazz, consider including those genres in your playlist. Second, it costs nothing and can be practiced anywhere. Music therapy has been widely studied and shown in numerous clinical trials to lower pain scores by several points [16].

There are several reasons why music therapy can help with pain. First, it functions as a passive distraction, reducing muscle tension. Music also helps lower anxiety, which in turn diminishes the perception of pain. Studies suggest listening to music for 30 minutes each day, or during times when pain is bothering you.

Massage

Massage is a therapeutic, hands-on treatment that harnesses the healing power of touch to relieve bodily pain. The power of touch emphasizes our fundamental need for connection and caring. Being touched by another person can be comforting and encourage healing.

Massage uses different levels of pressure to relax muscle tension and eliminate "knots," which are caused by tight muscle fibers that lead to pain. Additionally, massage alleviates pain by improving circulation and removing inflammatory waste products from the lymphatic system.

Many research studies have confirmed that massage therapy is effective for managing various types of cancer-related pain [17]. If you have peripheral neuropathy, and touch on the feet is not too intense, massage has also been found to benefit symptoms of neuropathy, even after only one treatment [18].

Aromatherapy

Aromatherapy might be one of the least recognized complementary therapies for pain. It involves diffusing plant-derived essential oils into the air and inhaling the mist indirectly. Most essential oils have a scent, and those commonly used for pain include peppermint, lavender, eucalyptus, rosemary, ginger, and clove. Simply choose the one that smells best to you and diffuse it nearby for 15–20 minutes daily, or for a longer period if you prefer.

Essential oils contain unique chemicals that, when inhaled, travel to the centers of the brain responsible for calming the nervous system. This calming effect alleviates pain. Like touch and music, smell is another of our senses that we can use to help our brains distract and disconnect from the experience of pain.

Aromatherapy has been shown to reduce pain from a breast biopsy [19], lower pain and anxiety after radiation and chemotherapy [20], and even reduce pain and the need for morphine at the end of life [21]. It is a safe and practical therapy, with no downsides.

Boswellia and Curcumin

Boswellia (frankincense) and curcumin (from turmeric root) are well-known for their powerful anti-inflammatory effects. They can be used individually or combined, and extensive research has explored how the two together support pain relief.

They have been found to help with digestive pain [22], pelvic pain [23], muscle pain [24], and joint pain [25]. As with any herbal medicine, safety is of utmost concern, and even at very high doses, the combination of these herbs does not appear to negatively affect liver, kidney, cholesterol, or blood parameters [26].

CLINICAL PEARL
Boswellia and curcumin both need to be taken in supplement form. Start with 300 mg each, two to three times per day.

Conclusion

As we bring this chapter to a close, you should now feel equipped with a diverse toolkit for pain management, one that extends far beyond conventional approaches. You've discovered how to actively engage your senses—whether it's through the comforting power of touch, the soothing sounds of music, or the therapeutic aromas of lavender and peppermint. You've also learned to harness the incredible power of your own body with exercise and to embrace the benefits of herbal medicine. You have taught yourself how to apply acupressure for an at-home treatment you can do anywhere. Managing pain can be an active, creative engagement with your entire being, empowering you to influence your comfort and well-being in unique, simple, and profound ways.

References

1 van den Beuken-van Everdingen MH, Hochstenbach LM, Joosten EA, et al. Update on prevalence of pain in patients with cancer: systematic review and meta-analysis. J Pain Symptom Manage, 2016; 51(1070–1090):e1079.

2 Wang L, Cohen JC, Devasenapathy N, et al. Prevalence and intensity of persistent post-surgical pain following breast cancer surgery: a systematic review and meta-analysis of observational studies. Br J Anaesth, 2020; 125(3):346–357.
3 Roberto A, Deandrea S, Greco MT, et al. Prevalence of neuropathic pain in cancer patients: pooled estimates from a systematic review of published literature and results from a survey conducted in 50 Italian palliative care centers. J Pain Symptom Manage, 2016; 51(6):1091–1102.
4 Sluka KA, Wager TD, Sutherland SP, et al. Predicting chronic postsurgical pain: current evidence and a novel program to develop predictive biomarker signatures. Pain, 2023; 164(9):1912–1926.
5 Zhenjie Y, Xiang Z. Electroacupuncture in the treatment of gastrointestinal dysfunction after laparoscopic nephrectomy: a retrospective analysis. BMC Complement Med Ther, 2025; 25(1):158.
6 Maurer J, Friedemann T, Chen Y, et al. A randomized controlled study on acupuncture for peri-operative pain after open radical prostatectomy. BJU Int, 2024; 133(6):725–732.
7 Lv JQ, Li PC, Zhou L, et al. Acupuncture at the P6 acupoint to prevent postoperative pain after craniotomy: a randomized, placebo-controlled study. Evid Based Complement Alternat Med, 2021; 2021: 6619855.
8 Lehky T, Fernandez IP, Krakow EF, et al. Neuropathy and muscle cramps in autologous and allogeneic hematopoietic cell transplantation survivors. Transplant Cell Therapy, 2022; 28(9):608.E1–608.E9.
9 Tian H, Luo Q, Huang L, et al. Exploration of the quantitative-effectiveness association between acupuncture temporal parameters and chemotherapy-induced peripheral neuropathy in cancer patients: a dose-response meta-analysis of randomized controlled trials. Front Oncol, 2025; 14:1527331.
10 Mao JJ, Ismaila N, Bao T, et al. Integrative medicine for pain management in oncology: society for integrative oncology-ASCO guidelines. J Clin Oncol, 40(34):3998–4024.
11 Zick SM, Sen A, Wyatt GK, et al. Investigation of 2 types of self-administered acupressure for persistent cancer-related fatigue in breast cancer survivors: a randomized clinical trial. JAMA Oncol, 2016; 2(11):1470–1476.
12 Zhao J, Zheng H, Wang X, et al. Efficacy of acupuncture in refractory irritable bowel syndrome patients: a randomized controlled trial. Front Med, 2024; 18(4):678–689.
13 Mechlińska A, Frąckiewicz K, Gładyś-Cieszyńska K, et al. Small intestinal bacterial overgrowth and intestinal methanogen overgrowth in gastrointestinal malignancies. Contemp Oncol, 2025; 29(1):11–21.
14 Peters M, Butson G, Mizrahi D, et al. Physical activity and pain in people with cancer: a systematic review and meta-analysis. Support Care Cancer, 2024; 32(3):145.

15 Toohey K, Hunter M, Paterson C, et al. Clinical updates on the effects of high intensity interval training (HIIT) exercise in people diagnosed with cancer: a systematic review and meta-analysis. J Sci Med Sport, 2023; 26(12):667–675.

16 Montoya LB, Mertilus DD. Decreasing pain intensity in adult patients with cancer through music therapy: a complementary non-pharmacoligical approach. Adv Pract Oncol, 2025; 16(2):57–64.

17 Win Myint O, Yoong SQ, Toh E, et al. Effectiveness of massage therapy for cancer pain, quality of life and anxiety levels: a systematic review and meta-analysis. J Clin Nurs, 2025; 34(1):49–87.

18 Yang M, Shao C, Shao C, et al. A retrospective cohort study on the preliminary efficacy of massage therapy for chemotherapy-induced peripheral neuropathy among cancer patients. Integr Cancer Ther, 2025; 24:15347354251323258.

19 Hancı E, Uslu Y, Arıbal E. The effect of aromatherapy on pain and anxiety levels before breast biopsy: a randomized controlled trial. Eur J Breast Health, 2025; 21(3):223–229.

20 Xie SR, Ma L, Xu XY. Effects of aromatherapy on physical and mental health of cancer patients undergoing radiotherapy and/or chemotherapy: a meta-analysis. Chin J Integr Med, 2024; 30(5):449–457.

21 Cullen G, Neely L, McDonald MR. The effect of aromatherapy in the management of cancer-related pain at the end of life: a pilot study. Clin J Oncol Nurs, 2023; 27(4):404–410.

22 Giacosa A, Riva A, Petrangolini G, et al. Beneficial effects on abdominal bloating with an innovative food-grade formulation of *Curcuma longa* and *Boswellia serrata* extracts in subjects with irritable bowel syndrome and small bowel dysbiosis. Nutrients, 2022; 14(3):416.

23 Presicce F, Barrese F, Cantiani A, et al. Boswellia resin extract and propolis derived polyphenols in patients with type III chronic prostatitis/chronic pelvic pain syndrome: an Italian prospective multicenter study. Asian J Urol, 2022; 9(2):139–145.

24 Rudrappa GH, Murthy M, Saklecha S, et al. Fast pain relief in exercise-induced acute musculoskeletal pain by turmeric-boswellia formulation: a randomized placebo-controlled double-blinded multicentre study. Medicine (Baltimore), 2022; 101(35):e30144.

25 Kumar B, Ghaytidak AB, Pandey AK, et al. A standardized *Boswellia serrata* extract improves knee joint function and cartilage morphology in human volunteers with mild to moderate osteoarthritis in a randomized placebo-controlled study. J Am Nutr Assoc, 2025; 44(5):375–386.

26 Kim SK, Jayachandran V, Vo TS, et al. Safety assessment of turmeric-boswellia-sesame formulation in healthy adult volunteers: an open-label prospective study. Adv Clin Exp Med, 2025; 34(8):1277–1288.

Part VI

Putting It All Together

16

The Six Foundations for Treating Cancer-related Fatigue

The way to get started is to quit talking and begin doing

—Walt Disney

You've embarked on a truly personal journey throughout this book, pausing at each reflection point to consider what truly resonated with you. By now, you've gathered a collection of powerful insights and recorded specific strategies you're eager to try. The goal has always been to help you craft a personalized fatigue management plan, one that's uniquely yours, that you can start putting into practice right away.

Remember, this isn't about finding a single magic bullet, but more about building a robust toolkit. If one approach doesn't quite hit the mark, you now have a wealth of other evidence-based therapies and ideas to explore, empowering you to continuously adapt and refine your path toward lasting energy.

To help you get started, some general recommendations for managing cancer-related fatigue are explained in Chapter 3. If you still don't know where to start, here is a step-by-step guide to help direct you.

Foundation 1—Comprehensive Blood Work

At the end of Chapter 2, a list of recommended blood work was provided. In the face of fatigue, a thorough laboratory workup is essential to help guide you toward the source of an obvious cause of low energy.

Beyond Cancer Fatigue: A Path to Reclaiming Energy, First Edition. Jessa Landmann, ND.

Source of fatigue	Recommended blood work	Next steps
Thyroid dysfunction	TSH, fT4, fT3, anti-TPO, anti-TG	If abnormal, see Chapter 5.
Anemia	Ferritin, transferrin saturation, ESR, complete blood cell count, vitamin B12, folate	Low iron, vitamin B12, and folate can be supplemented. See Chapter 7. If transferrin saturation is less than 20%, with high ferritin, anemia of chronic disease is likely, and you must lower inflammation with any strategies recommended in this book. Start with Chapter 4 on Nutrition.
Stress	4-Point cortisol, or AM cortisol	If cortisol is high, see Chapter 12 on Stress and Anxiety.
Blood sugar imbalance	Fasting insulin, fasting glucose, HbA1C.	If elevated, see Chapter 8 on Diabetes.
Inflammation	C-reactive protein, neutrophil-to-lymphocyte ratio	If high, you must take steps to lower inflammation. Every therapy in this book lowers inflammation. See any chapter that feels most relevant to you.

Foundation 2—Nutrition

Nutrition is not just about what we eat, but also how much. We've discussed nutrition throughout this book, and a good place to start to ensure you're getting the optimal combination of inflammation-lowering, high-protein foods is the Mediterranean Diet. Refer to Chapter 9 on Weight Loss for the food pyramid and recommended serving sizes. At the bare minimum, your daily goals are five to six servings of fruits and vegetables, 20 g of fiber, two to three servings of healthy fats, and ample protein. Refer to Chapter 4 on Nutrition for guidance on serving sizes and for a discussion on the best foods and eating patterns for increasing energy.

In Chapter 9, you learned how to calculate your basal metabolic rate, giving you a clear understanding of your ideal calorie intake. This helps you fuel your body effectively without overdoing it. Then, to directly support your energy goals, Chapter 17 is packed with practical meal ideas designed to help you easily hit your daily protein targets. These meals are designed to provide your body with the sustained energy it needs to thrive.

Ultimately, for your energy to truly soar, consistent, proper nourishment is non-negotiable. It's the essential fuel your body needs to thrive.

Foundation 3—Physical Activity

If you're not moving your body regularly, your energy will never truly reach its peak potential. We hope the previous chapters have already sparked your curiosity, perhaps inspiring you to try yoga, lift weights, or explore the gentle flow of Tai chi. The consistent message throughout this book is simple: the type of physical activity matters far less than simply engaging in something you genuinely enjoy and something that makes your body feel strong and alive.

To build a reserve of lasting energy, Chapter 18 will guide you on how to start building muscle. For tailored exercise guidance, including specific durations if you're managing blood sugar imbalances, Chapter 8 provides clear instructions and a wealth of enjoyable activities. Feel free to revisit these chapters for inspiration and practical advice.

If you're a cancer survivor struggling with fatigue and you're not yet moving your body most days, this is the first place to start. Physical activity is one of the most impactful and inspiring steps you can take to reclaim your energy and vitality.

Foundation 4—Sleep

We all know sleep is essential, but for truly sustained energy, it's a cornerstone. That's why Chapter 14 is one of the longest in this book, packed with numerous scientifically backed strategies to help you achieve truly restorative sleep.

While those proven techniques are crucial, it's also vital to identify if anything else is hijacking your rest. Issues like pain, restless legs, or hot flashes can severely disrupt sleep, and Chapters 6 and 15 offer solutions for managing these symptoms.

Your goal should be to aim for seven to eight hours of quality sleep each night. While individual needs can vary, if you're experiencing persistent daytime sleepiness, it's worth considering sleep apnea as a potential cause of that relentless fatigue. Prioritizing your sleep should be one of the first steps you take.

Foundation 5—Mental and Emotional Health

Neglecting our thoughts and feelings is one of the biggest mistakes we can make when it comes to replenishing our energy levels. It's a direct path to feeling perpetually drained. Our mental and emotional states aren't just "in our heads" as you have learned, but rather, they profoundly impact our physical energy.

When your brain works overtime, it constantly releases stress hormones that interfere with sleep, disrupt digestion, and even fuel inflammation—all major energy drains. When your emotional battery is constantly running on empty from these internal battles, your physical energy simply can't flourish.

That's why nurturing your mental and emotional health is a foundation. Chapters 11–13 address depression, anxiety, stress, and fear of recurrence. Utilize the strategies in those chapters to unburden yourself from the constant demands of emotional distress, helping you to get rid of fatigue, once and for all.

Foundation 6 – Spiritual Connection

Beyond the physical and emotional, there lies an untapped source of energy in spiritual connection. This isn't necessarily about organized religion, but rather about connecting to something larger than oneself—whether it's nature, a sense of purpose, community, or an inner belief system. In the face of a challenging diagnosis like cancer, and during the often arduous journey of survivorship, this connection can become an essential foundation for mental, emotional, and even physical resilience, profoundly impacting your energy levels.

A spiritual connection may be found through breath work, yoga, or meditation, and offers a unique kind of replenishment. It can also be found through a gratitude practice or by serving others. It can provide a sense of meaning and purpose, even amidst suffering, helping to shift focus from what's lost to what can still be found. This sense of meaning can ignite a quiet but powerful energy that sustains you through difficult moments. Furthermore, spiritual practices often foster feelings of hope, peace, and acceptance, which are powerful antidotes to anxiety, fear, and sadness. This sense of peace and purpose translates into a sustained sense of energy.

Conclusion

Your energy may not be something that just returns to you from lost depths. It is a cultivated outcome meticulously built upon the six aforementioned foundations. Each choice you make in these areas is a powerful step toward not just managing fatigue, but also reigniting your very best self.

17

A Fatigue-fighting Meal Plan

One cannot think well, love well or sleep well, if one has not dined well

—Virginia Woolf

Let's put all this fantastic nutrition knowledge into action! In this chapter, we delve into practical ways to create energy-boosting meals.

The Power of a Balanced Plate

Throughout this book, we've explored the essential macronutrients: protein, carbohydrates, and healthy fats—all crucial for providing the energy your body needs. We've also highlighted foods rich in fiber, iron, and vitamin B12, which are well-known for their energy-boosting properties. Remember our discussions on the importance of anti-inflammatory foods and how those vibrant, colorful additions to your plate can help reduce inflammation. We also learned that restrictive diets often aren't the answer, especially when fatigue is a concern. Instead, the key to sustained energy lies in a balanced plate packed with nutrient-dense foods.

Your Fuel for Fatigue: Protein and Calories

To effectively fight fatigue, your meal plan should be rich in antioxidants, high in fiber, and most importantly, high in protein. Protein is essential, especially as we age, to maintain muscle mass. This helps you stay strong, balanced, and full of both physical and mental energy. It's surprisingly common for people, particularly women, to not get enough protein. This chapter is designed to offer you inspiring ideas to help you achieve your protein targets. Think of it as a friendly

Beyond Cancer Fatigue: A Path to Reclaiming Energy, First Edition. Jessa Landmann, ND.

guide to spark your creativity and help you discover delicious ways to incorporate more protein into your daily routine.

Additionally, earlier in the book, you calculated your basal metabolic rate. This is the number of calories you need to consume to support basic bodily functions and ensure your body receives the energy it requires. You must confirm through food tracking that you are consuming enough calories. Healthy fats and complex carbohydrates help you achieve this. That is why, in the suggested meal plans, not only is the protein content calculated, but also the carbohydrates, fats, and total calories.

Calculating Your Protein Needs

As a quick reminder, here's how to calculate your daily protein target: take your weight in kilograms and multiply it by 1.2–1.5. The result is the amount of protein in grams you should aim for each day. You'll be amazed at how easily you can meet this goal by selecting just three to four of the meal ideas, smoothies, and snacks provided in this chapter.

Have fun experimenting, and enjoy discovering your favorite new high-protein meals!

Breakfast: The Foundation for Energy

You know that feeling when you're ready to hit the ground running, full of energy for the day ahead? Well, maybe it's been a while since you felt that way, but breakfast is your secret weapon for that! It's like giving your body a gentle nudge to wake up its metabolism and providing the steady fuel you need. Some people say they aren't hungry in the morning and prefer to eat later. However, from your body's perspective, it has been "fasting" all night while you slept, so it's naturally eager to refuel and get going. If you do not like breakfast and are persistently fatigued, training yourself to become a "breakfast of champions" person is highly recommended.

Why Your Body Loves a Morning Meal

You've learned that cortisol should naturally be at its highest in the morning. If it doesn't reach this peak, low morning cortisol levels can contribute to low energy throughout the day. One way to boost your cortisol in the morning is by eating. Studies have shown that people who regularly skip breakfast tend to have lower cortisol levels in the morning [1]. Having a high cortisol level in the morning wakes up your metabolism, which helps with weight management.

Steady Energy with No Crashes

Beyond cortisol, studies also show that a good morning meal has a fantastic impact on your blood sugar. It helps keep it steady, preventing those frustrating energy crashes that can leave you feeling utterly drained by midmorning or afternoon. Having breakfast may also prevent diabetes and metabolic syndrome [2].

So, to truly set yourself up for a day packed with steady energy, aim for a breakfast that's rich in protein, includes satisfying complex carbohydrates, and is low in highly processed foods. When you give your body a nutrient-dense, energy-packed meal to start the day, it's an investment in feeling your best!

Option 1: Egg White Omelet With Feta, Peppers, and Tomatoes with Berries

The protein in eggs is in the white part; therefore, crack the eggs into a measuring cup and remove the yolks to get an accurate measurement. If you prefer a bit more richness, leave a yolk or two. If you don't like feta cheese, you can substitute cheddar or skip the cheese altogether. The cheese adds a bit more protein and flavor. The vegetables provide an antioxidant-rich, inflammation-lowering boost, complemented by the blueberries on the side.

Ingredients	Nutrition content	327 calories
1 cup egg white	Protein	41 g
1/4 cup crumbled feta cheese	Carbohydrate	20 g
5 cherry tomatoes	Fats	8 g
1/2 chopped orange pepper	Fiber	3 g
1 cup spinach	Iron	17 mg
1/2 cup blueberries		

Option 2: Cottage Cheese with Berries and Pumpkin Seeds

If weight loss is a goal, consider opting for nonfat cottage cheese. If weight recovery is a goal, then full-fat or regular cottage cheese may be a better option. Cottage cheese and pumpkin seeds are excellent sources of protein, and the fruit adds the extra antioxidants you need.

Ingredients	Nutrition content	251 calories
1/2 cup nonfat cottage cheese	Protein	17 g
1 oz pumpkin seeds	Carbohydrate	17 g
1/2 cup raspberries	Fats	15 g
	Fiber	7 g
	Iron	17 mg

Option 3: Protein Pancakes

Smash a banana, add two eggs, and a half scoop of whey protein powder (vanilla or chocolate works best). Cook the pancake in a pan as you normally would. Whey protein powder is the best for maintaining muscle mass as it is considered a complete protein and contains all of the amino acids you need for muscle recovery and growth.

Ingredients	Nutrition content	350 calories
1 banana	Protein	27 g
2 eggs	Carbohydrate	28 g
1/2 scoop whey protein powder	Fats	10 g
	Fiber	3 g
	Iron	11 mg

Option 4: Breakfast Wrap

Scramble the eggs first, then add salt and pepper to taste. Next, mix in the beans and tomatoes to soften and warm them. Pile the mixture on top of a tortilla, add the cheese to melt, and roll into a wrap. One egg provides about 6 g of protein; therefore, finding ways to incorporate more protein, such as through beans or cheese, is a little trick to make a more protein-packed breakfast.

Ingredients	Nutrition content	466 calories
2 eggs scrambled	Protein	27 g
1 flour tortilla	Carbohydrate	35 g
5 cherry tomatoes	Fats	23 g
1/4 cup black beans	Fiber	6 g
1 oz cheddar cheese	Iron	33 mg

Option 5: Oatmeal with a Twist

Cook the oatmeal as you normally would, adding the spices to the water and oats, and add the toppings afterward. The peanut butter adds some extra protein, as plant-based breakfasts, such as oatmeal, are generally lower in protein. However, with the carbohydrate intake from the berries and oats, and healthy fats from the walnuts, this oatmeal will keep you full for hours.

Ingredients	Nutrition content	491 calories
1/2 cup oats	Protein	13 g
1/8 tsp cinnamon	Carbohydrate	41 g
1/8 tsp cardamom	Fats	32 g
1 tbsp peanut butter	Fiber	8 g
1/4 cup blueberries	Iron	17 mg
1/4 cup walnuts		
1 tbsp shredded coconut		

Option 6: Hummus and Avocado Toast

Smash the avocado, adding lime juice, salt, and pepper to taste. Layer the toast first with hummus, then avocado, and top with the fried eggs. If you wish to make this vegetarian, skip the eggs and try some grilled tofu on top for extra protein.

Ingredients	Nutrition content	427 calories
2 fried eggs	Protein	18 g
1 tbsp hummus	Carbohydrate	29 g
1/2 avocado	Fats	25 g
1 slice whole grain toast	Fiber	8 g
	Iron	11 mg

With 3 oz of grilled tofu, the protein content is 15 g.

Option 7: Yogurt Bowl with Nuts and Berries

Greek yogurt is high in protein, and the nuts and berries provide anti-inflammatory, healthy fats, and antioxidants that help lower inflammation and increase energy.

Ingredients	Nutrition content	259 calories
3/4 cup Greek Yogurt	Protein	19 g
1.5 ounces almonds	Carbohydrate	29 g
1/2 cup strawberries	Fats	7 g
	Fiber	4 g
	Iron	6 mg

Lunch: Replenishing Energy Stores

Depending on whom you speak to, some nutrition consultants recommend eating several small meals throughout the day to maintain high energy levels, but this approach may lead to overeating and potentially contribute to weight gain. The goal of these meal plan ideas is for each meal to provide ample energy from calories, complex carbohydrates, and protein, so you feel energized between meals. With lunch ideas, focus on lean proteins, plenty of chunky filling vegetables, and healthy carbohydrates.

Why the recommendation for chunky vegetables, you may be wondering? Chunky vegetables are those that require thorough chewing to swallow without risk of choking. Examples of chunky vegetables include broccoli, carrots, peppers, cucumbers, cauliflower, and sweet potatoes. Including foods like this in our diet forces us to chew for more extended periods, and we also tend to eat more slowly. Chewing and eating slowly causes us to feel fuller, which helps prevent weight gain [3]. Slow chewing also increases blood flow to the gut, which aids digestion [4].

Option 1: Chunky Greek Salad with Grilled Chicken

This is a modified Greek salad, omitting feta cheese, but feel free to add it if you prefer. Grill the chicken on a barbecue or in the oven, preparing it to your liking. Add the chicken to a bowl of chopped veggies and olive oil.

Ingredients	Nutrition content	320 calories
4 oz grilled chicken	Protein	23 g
1/2 cup chopped peppers	Carbohydrate	15 g
1/2 cup cherry tomatoes	Fats	24 g
1 chopped mini cucumber	Fiber	3 g

Ingredients	Nutrition content	320 calories
7–10 olives, chopped	Iron	7 mg
1 tbsp olive oil		

Option 2: Tuna Pasta Salad

Canned tuna is an excellent way to get protein if you don't have much time to cook. Mixing it with some whole wheat pasta and greens provides a hearty meal with a clean dressing.

Ingredients	Nutrition content	432 calories
I can flaked tuna	Protein	40 g
1 cup cooked whole wheat pasta	Carbohydrate	42 g
1 cup spinach	Fats	11 g
1 tbsp hemp seeds	Fiber	6 g
1/2 lemon, juiced	Iron	23 mg
1 tsp olive oil		

Option 3: Lentil Quinoa Medley

For vegetarian options when meat or fish might not be what we crave, the trick to high-protein meals is to combine grains and legumes. Add some vegetables and your preferred dressing. An easy go-to dressing can be made from lemon juice, olive oil, and garlic. Challenge yourself with other homemade dressings.

Ingredients	Nutrition content	368 calories
1/2 cup cooked lentils	Protein	14 g
1/2 cup cooked quinoa	Carbohydrate	44 g
1/2 cup chopped parsley	Fats	15 g
1/2 cup chopped broccoli, raw or steamed	Fiber	12 g
1 minced garlic, 1 squeezed lemon, and 1 tbsp olive oil for dressing	Iron	29 mg

Option 4: Shredded Chicken Rainbow Salad

Dark meat is richer in iron than white meat and is often more palatable for people. Shred the meat and vegetables, tossing them into a mixture. Mix the dressing, and sprinkle the mint on top.

Ingredients	Nutrition content	312 calories
4 oz shredded chicken thigh	Protein	27 g
2 carrots, shredded	Carbohydrate	19 g
1/2 pepper, cut in strips	Fat	14 g
1/2 cucumber, julienned	Fiber	5 g
Handful arugula	Iron	12 mg
Mint chopped		
2 tbsp soy sauce, 1 squeezed lime, 1/8 tsp ginger, 2 tsp olive oil for dressing		

Option 5: Simple Grilled Chicken Club

Roasting a chicken or cooking a few chicken breasts in advance is always a smart move—you'll have an easy source of protein ready to slice or chop for sandwiches, wraps, or salads. Add 4 oz of chicken breast to your favorite whole-grain bread, add some toppings, and voila!

Ingredients	Nutrition content	203 calories
4 oz grilled chicken	Protein	25 g
Butterleaf lettuce	Carbohydrate	18 g
1/2 slice tomato	Fats	4 g
Handful broccoli sprouts	Fiber	3 g
1 tbsp Dijon mustard	Iron	9 mg
2 slices rye bread		

Dinner: Finishing the Day Strong

In reality, the recipes for lunch and dinner are interchangeable, but it is still essential to ensure that both meals are high in protein. High protein intake in the evening helps promote restful sleep and supports muscle maintenance while we sleep. As the third meal of the day, it's a great chance to include anything that may have been lacking earlier, such as more fiber or healthy fats. As discussed elsewhere in the book, try not to eat too late in the evening, and aim to finish dinner at least three to four hours before you usually go to bed.

Option 1: Maple Turkey Burgers with Roasted Green Beans and Carrots

Mix the turkey, maple syrup, and herbs in a bowl, and divide the mixture into four patties. In a separate bowl, combine the tamari, sesame oil, and sesame seeds, then toss in the vegetables. Roast the vegetables at 400 °F for 20 minutes while you grill the burgers.

Ingredients	Nutrition content	420 calories
1 lb Extra Lean Ground Turkey	Protein	21 g per patty
1 cup chopped carrots and green bean	Carbohydrate	25 g
2 tbsp maple syrup	Fats	19 g
1 tsp thyme	Fiber	6 g
1 tsp sage	Iron	4 mg
Salt and pepper		
Veggies marinade: 2 tbsp each tamari, sesame oil, and sesame seeds		

Option 2: Red Curry Salmon with Vegetables

Healthy fats are beneficial for the brain and can help improve mood, making this delicious dish an excellent choice for leaving you feeling happy and content. In a mildly heated pan, add the coconut milk and red curry paste, stirring to blend. Add the salmon filet and steam it for six to nine minutes, adding the veggies and edamame in the last two minutes. Serve over rice if you like.

Ingredients	Nutrition content	300 calories
4 oz salmon filet	Protein	30 g
1/2 cup coconut milk	Carbohydrate	14 g
1 tbsp red curry paste	Fats	13 g
1 cup chopped bok choy	Fiber	4 g
1/2 red pepper	Iron	23 mg
1/4 cup edamame beans		

Option 3: Shrimp Tacos

Tacos are a convenient dinner option, and shrimp are surprisingly high in protein, helping to keep you full. You can add anything you want to tacos, but here is one idea for you. Sprinkle the paprika over the shrimp, and cook in a pan for a few minutes, adding the peppers in the last minute. Spoon the shrimp over the tortillas, topping with avocado and cilantro.

Ingredients	Nutrition content	348 calories
4 oz shrimp	Protein	22 g
1/2 tsp paprika	Carbohydrate	34 g
2 mini corn tortillas	Fats	15 g
1/2 yellow pepper, chopped	Fiber	7 g
1/2 avocado, diced	Iron	4 mg
Cilantro to sprinkle on top		

Option 4: Penne with Chickpeas and Burst Tomatoes

When preparing vegetarian dishes, it's always a good idea to pair grains with legumes to maximize protein content. Prepare the penne noodles, and in the meantime, heat the tomatoes, garlic, olive oil, salt, and pepper in a pan until all the tomatoes have burst. In the last minute, heat the chickpeas in the sauce, spoon over the noodles, and top with fresh basil.

Ingredients	Nutrition content	347 calories
1 cup cooked whole wheat noodles	Protein	15 g
4 oz chickpeas	Carbohydrate	65 g
2 cups cherry tomatoes	Fats	8 g
2 garlic cloves	Fiber	11 g
Basil to sprinkle on top	Iron	20 mg

Option 5: Classic Chicken Stir-fry

Stir-fry dishes are amazing because you can add whatever you have in your fridge. Start with a gentle sauté of garlic and ginger, then pour in chicken broth and soy sauce to steam your preferred vegetables. Finally, heat the cooked chicken for the last minute. Pour over rice and enjoy.

Ingredients	Nutrition content	476 calories
4 oz cooked chicken	Protein	39 g
2 cups chopped veggies (broccoli, carrots, snow peas, peppers)	Carbohydrate	60 g
1/2 cup chicken broth	Fats	10 g
1/3 cup soy sauce	Fiber	9 g
2 garlic cloves, chopped	Iron	22 mg
1 tsp ginger, chopped		
1/2 cup brown rice		

Sustaining Snacks

In between meals, we may need a little pick-me-up. Snacks are okay during the day, but keep your choices consistent with the messages of this book, especially to boost energy. Have some fruit with nuts, or veggies and hummus. Have sliced apples dipped in almond butter, or some Greek yogurt with berries. Avoid reaching for junk foods and boxed snacks from stores, as they can decrease our energy levels. Another great midday snack is a high-protein smoothie to boost your energy.

Smoothie Recipes

Never underestimate the role of the good old-fashioned smoothie. You can pack a lot in a smoothie to make it a power-packed on-the-go drink. Buy a chocolate, vanilla, or unflavored whey protein powder, and add one scoop to each smoothie.

Most protein powders are approximately 25 g of protein per scoop. As you learned in Chapter 10, whey protein is the protein of choice for putting on and sustaining muscle. Add other ingredients as desired to suit your taste preferences. If the smoothies are too thick, add water. Here are some delicious starting points!

Option 1: Classic Berry and Banana

- 3/4 cup frozen berries, 1/2 banana, whey protein powder, 1 cup almond milk.

Option 2: Tropical Green Smoothie

- 1 cup frozen pineapple, 1 cup spinach, 2 tbsp hemp seeds, whey protein powder, 1 cup almond milk.

Option 3: Blueberry Detox

- 1 cup frozen blueberries, 2 kale leaves, 1 tbsp ground flax, whey protein powder, 1.5 cups water.

Option 4: Chocolate Cauliflower Concoction

- 1 banana, 1/2 cup cauliflower, 1 tbsp peanut butter, 1 tbsp cocoa powder, whey protein powder, 1 cup water, 1/2 cup coconut milk.

Option 5: Mango Oat Smoothie

- 1 cup frozen mango, 1/2 banana, 1/4 cup oats, 1 tbsp hemp seeds, whey protein powder, 1.5 cups almond milk.

Conclusion

These recipe ideas are designed to be simple to prepare, allowing anyone to make them. They are high-energy meals because they contain a healthy balance of calories, protein, healthy fats, and carbs. Eating is a personal choice, and the style of eating mentioned above might not suit everyone. If you don't like the recipes listed, look for cookbooks or websites that focus on high-protein, Mediterranean-style cooking, as this is the most effective way to maintain energy over the long term.

At the end of the day, nutrition isn't just about food—it's one of the most powerful foundations of your health and a primary source of creating lasting energy.

References

1 Chawla S, Beretoulis S, Deere A, et al. The window matters: a systematic review of time restricted eating strategies in relation to cortisol and melatonin secretion. Nutrients, 2021; 13(8):2525.
2 Odegaard AO, Jacobs Jr DR, Steffen LM, et al. Breakfast frequency and development of metabolic risk. Diabetes Care, 2013; 36:3100–3106.
3 Ohkuma T, Hirakawa Y, Nakamura U, et al. Association between eating rate and obesity: a systematic review and meta-analysis. Int J Obes (Lond), 2015; 39:1589–1596.
4 Hamada Y, Kashima H, Hayashi N. The number of chews and meal duration affect diet-induced thermogenesis and splanchnic circulation. Obesity (Silver Spring), 2014; 22:E62–E69.

18

How to Build a Booty

As we develop our physical muscles through overcoming opposition—such as lifting weights—we develop our character muscles by overcoming challenges and adversity

—Stephen Covey

Years may wrinkle the skin, but to give up enthusiasm wrinkles the soul

—Samuel Ullman

Many might see aging as slowing down, but what if you could create a reserve of strength and vitality that defies this narrative? The key lies in an overlooked organ system: your muscles. Far from being solely about strength and appearance, your muscles are a powerhouse that impacts your energy, brain health, and overall ability to thrive as the years go by.

Apart from aging, cancer survivors often lose muscle mass during treatment, especially if they don't stay active. Depending on your age and activity level at diagnosis, being older and less active increases the risk of greater muscle loss. Your muscles are involved in everything, from how your body uses fuel to how restful your sleep is. Having a strong muscular system is the best foundation for sustained energy and a vibrant life.

Why Muscle Matters More Than You Think

Throughout this book, you may have noticed that every chapter recommends some form of physical activity as a treatment. Regular exercise supports your thyroid health by helping lower cortisol and boost T3 and T4 levels. It can also sharpen your focus and memory, helping to combat "chemo brain." Exercise is

Beyond Cancer Fatigue: A Path to Reclaiming Energy, First Edition. Jessa Landmann, ND.

a key player in weight management and blood sugar control, especially for those with diabetes or pre-diabetes.

Beyond that, it's a proven way to get better sleep, reduce pain, and ease symptoms of depression and anxiety. Overall, it is one of the most valuable investments you can make for your cancer recovery and long-term energy and well-being.

Muscle is known to support our physical stability and mobility, and prevent falls as we age. Less muscle may mean more fat content, which puts us at a higher risk of being overweight and developing cardiovascular issues. More fat and less muscle also lead to greater inflammation, as muscle has been shown to increase antioxidant enzymes and reduce overall inflammation [1].

Lower muscle mass puts you at a higher risk of dementia and speeds the rate of cognitive decline in those developing dementia [2]. Low muscle mass is one of the strongest predictors of a loss of independence as you age [3].

If you ever have to have a surgery or are hospitalized, low muscle mass puts you at a higher risk of infections, surgical complications, and longer hospital stays. If you ever require more cancer treatment, low muscle mass is associated with worse side effects of chemotherapy [4] and possibly a worse response to treatment [5]. Low muscle mass may even predict long-term survival in those with cancer [6, 7].

Low muscle mass may also be associated with an increased risk of cancer development. Studies have found that over 50% of cancer patients have low muscle mass at the time of diagnosis [8]. One reason this could be is the consistent observation that physical inactivity is a risk factor for cancer in the first place.

This book is dedicated to helping cancer survivors regain energy and overcome fatigue. The reality is this: if you are not engaging in physical activity, you are missing a crucial part of the puzzle. Without activity, you lose muscle mass, which can worsen sleep, slow down your metabolism, lead to weight gain, and decrease your mood, confidence, and overall quality of life.

It's time to get honest about it, and it's time to get excited about it. Regular exercise is one of the greatest gifts you can give to yourself.

The Lies We Tell Ourselves

The most common reasons people give for not exercising are a lack of time, energy, and motivation. Other barriers include boredom, not enjoying the activity, low confidence in one's abilities, fear of injury, limited support from a partner, financial constraints, and transportation challenges.

Time

This is one of the biggest lies you tell yourself. It's not that you don't have time; it's that you haven't made it a priority. If you genuinely feel you don't have time, jot down your activities on a piece of paper or another device for a week. Identify times when you may be idle, and find at least three 30-minute blocks each week to dedicate to physical activity. Idle time is often spent watching TV, surfing the internet, napping during the day, or traveling to and from appointments.

Find ways to make use of this idle time. Can you walk or cycle between appointments? Can you stand while using the computer? Can you swap the TV for a walk? Instead of napping, can you attend a fitness class?

Energy

It's completely normal to feel like the last thing you want to do when you're tired is exercise. Yet, the incredible truth is that moving your body is one of the most powerful ways to create more energy! The key is to truly believe that physical activity, even in small doses, will make you feel better.

Don't hesitate to start with something as simple as five sit-ups, a quick five-minute walk, or a few stretches. Starting when you're already feeling drained can feel daunting, so the secret is to avoid pushing too hard, especially if you haven't been active for a while.

There is power in taking small steps. Think about learning something new, like a language or an instrument. Did you start by debating complex topics in French, or did you begin by counting to ten? Did you tackle a Mozart concerto on day one, or did you learn "Twinkle, Twinkle Little Star"? Just like those experiences, building an exercise habit means starting small and being consistent. Every little bit of movement adds up, helping you build momentum and gradually discover the incredible energy boost that comes from moving your body.

Motivation

You've already learned so much about the incredible power of exercise. How it can dramatically improve your quality of life, help manage treatment side effects, and why maintaining muscle is so vital. But if you're still finding it tough to get started, remember that motivation often follows action, rather than preceding it. You can't wait for motivation to strike—you have to create it!

Invite a friend to join you on this fitness adventure. Having someone to share the journey with can make all the difference, offering accountability and a boost of shared encouragement.

Or take a few moments each day to practice guided imagery. Close your eyes and vividly imagine yourself enjoying exercise, and truly visualize yourself brimming with boundless energy. Let that feeling pull you forward.

Lack of Skill

Many activities require no special skills, such as walking, climbing stairs, jogging, hiking, doing push-ups, sitting and standing from a chair, or dancing around your kitchen. Shooting hoops at a basketball court, kicking a soccer ball, or riding a stationary bike also don't need skill training. Nervous about lifting weights? Most exercise machines at a gym have instructions on how to use them, and if you're still unsure, ask a staff member for help.

Having a lack of skill is a lie you tell yourself, which is a mental barrier. You need to start telling yourself that you have the skills to do most types of physical exercise. Of course, for some new activities, like skiing, a lesson may be recommended, but you do not have to spend money on lessons of any kind. And most importantly, you do not need to acquire any new skills.

Boredom

This is simple—avoid activities you find boring. If jogging or yoga isn't interesting to you, that's okay. There are plenty of other options you can try. Surely, there's at least one thing you can enjoy doing.

Cost and Transportation

You can already see how most activities can be done free of charge. You do not need an expensive gym membership, nor do you need to pay for expensive lessons. You do not need a car to drive to a fitness center, as many of the activities listed above can be done at home or in a park.

REFLECTION POINT

Recognize what prevents you from staying active regularly. Write down any lies you tell yourself and apply CBT techniques you've learned elsewhere in this book to reframe your self-talk.

Do you tell yourself you don't have time? Instead, try saying to yourself, "I will find 30 minutes per day to exercise, as I am a person who prioritizes my health and energy."

What other obstacles do you face in your life that prevent you from exercising regularly? Is child care an issue? If so, could you swap babysitting with a friend to find time? Or are there exercises you can do while the kids are with you, such as skipping rope?

Spend some time reflecting on this topic, and figure out ways to overcome your obstacles.

How to Build a Booty

While conditioning and strengthening all the major muscles in your body is important, for someone just starting with an exercise routine, it can be helpful to focus on one major muscle group to set you up for success.

The major muscle that makes up your backside is the gluteus maximus, the largest muscle in the body. The other muscles of the upper leg, the quadriceps and hamstrings, are also large muscles that get involved when you're trying to build muscle in the butt. Because these muscles are large, they respond very quickly to exercise, allowing you to see and feel rapid results.

If you have historically been active and regularly participate in physical exercise, whether through sport or other gym activities, then definitely keep doing the activities you enjoy. For those who are just beginning or returning to activity after a long period of muscle inactivity, this section will help you get started.

Over time, you should start to involve other muscles, like the back, biceps, and calves. However, after many years of clinical experience, this method of working on the glutes to quickly build muscle has been successful in directly increasing energy levels, helping people feel stronger, and creating motivation to persevere on their fitness journey.

Here are your instructions on how to build a booty!

First, Assess Your Readiness for Weight Lifting, and If Necessary, Seek Out a Doctor

Generally speaking, the exercises that follow are safe to perform and do not require a doctor's clearance to get started. However, if you have serious cardiovascular complications, it is always essential to consult with a physician who is qualified and experienced in physical activity counseling.

When lifting weights, there can sometimes be increased pressure in the abdomen. If you have an ostomy bag, seeking extra guidance in this area might be helpful. Additionally, if you have bone metastases, extra caution is necessary, and consulting a healthcare professional is recommended.

If you have injuries that you need to work around, most personal trainers or other fitness professionals should be able to provide a proper assessment to help you manage them effectively. They will evaluate your overall health, identify any potential limitations, and offer personalized guidance based on your medical history, if necessary.

You can also self-evaluate your physical readiness by completing the Physical Activity Readiness Questionnaire (PAR-Q). This is available online for free and can be filled out independently, helping you understand the key considerations for assessing the safety of starting an exercise program.

Second, Listen to Your Body

If you are not currently active, it is wise to start at a slower and more leisurely pace than you might expect. Remember the analogy about learning a new language: it's easier to begin with counting than discussing politics. If you experience knee or back pain, you may need to be more cautious about which exercises require modifications. Always seek professional advice to ensure you perform all exercises safely and with injury prevention in mind.

As humans, our brains tend to be impatient and seek quick results. However, doing "too much too soon" can lead to an injury. Engaging in an activity that is too intense or too long can actually make you feel more tired. A general rule of thumb is that exercise should leave you feeling invigorated afterward; if you feel wiped out, you've done too much.

Always remember to warm up and cool down, and rest between activity days. Most importantly, pay attention to pain. Pain is your body's stop signal, especially after a cancer diagnosis.

Third, Stay Consistent

Consistency is essential for reaching your fitness goals. Aim for at least three to four strength training sessions each week, lasting 20–30 minutes, with rest days in between. On rest days, gentle movement such as yoga, walking, or stretching routines is recommended. Staying consistent is the key to noticing progress.

Fourth, Fuel Your Body

Muscle growth occurs when muscle-building processes exceed muscle breakdown. To achieve this, the muscles must work against resistance—such as lifting weights—and the body needs enough fuel, particularly from protein and carbohydrates, to support recovery and growth.

Aim to eat a high-protein meal within an hour after your workout. While both plant-based and animal-based diets can support muscle growth, research shows that the greatest gains typically come from animal proteins [9]. If you follow a primarily plant-based diet, it's especially important to ensure you're eating enough calories to support muscle building. Adding whey protein powder to smoothies is an easy way to boost your protein intake.

Carbohydrates are also crucial after a weight-lifting workout. Carbs stimulate the hormone insulin, which is a trigger for muscle growth and helps transport protein into the muscle. By combining carbs with protein within 30 minutes of weightlifting, muscle growth may increase by up to 145% [10].

Fifth, Be Patient and Enjoy the Journey

Building strength and muscle takes time and effort. Don't get discouraged by slow progress. Celebrate your achievements, enjoy the process, and remember that every journey begins with a single step. However, if you follow the exercises below and ensure you eat a high-protein, high-carbohydrate meal after weightlifting, you should see quick results.

This chapter provides a foundational framework for your weightlifting journey. Remember to prioritize safety, consistency, and proper form. By following these guidelines, you'll be well on your way to experiencing the numerous benefits of resistance training.

Exercises

If you are new to exercise or haven't worked out in a while, do each exercise using only your body weight. When body weight exercises become too easy and your muscles no longer feel sore or tired, gradually add heavier weights. Resistance bands are excellent tools for providing resistance and can be placed above the knees for each of the following exercises.

To build muscle, the last two to three repetitions should be difficult. When they become easy, you need to increase resistance. You can hold dumbbells, heavy water bottles, or bags of groceries. The key is to keep adding heavier weights to ensure your muscles remain challenged, as this is how they grow.

All exercises should start with 15 repetitions, three times. Do this routine three times per week.

1. Squats—Considered to be a basic move for building glutes. Stand with your legs about shoulder-width apart, toes slightly turned out. Lower down to a deep squat, and stand up, squeezing the glutes. Start with body weight, and progress to holding weights.

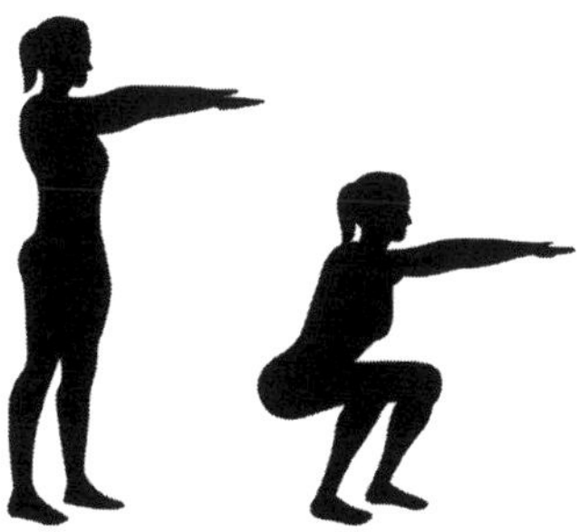

2. Leg Extension—This can be done while standing or lying on your stomach. It's a good exercise to perform with an exercise band, especially around the ankles or knees. Ensure that you don't arch your back, focusing solely on the glutes.

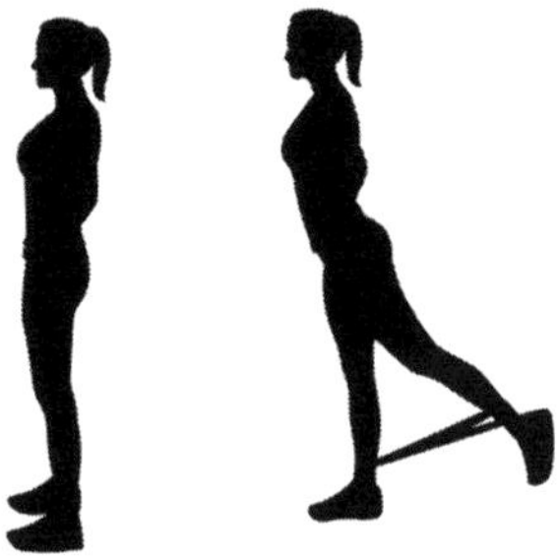

3. Step Up—At home, this can be done onto one stair, two stairs for more of a challenge, or onto a chair. Focus on keeping your knee aligned straight forward and contracting your glutes. Start with body weight, and progress to holding weights.

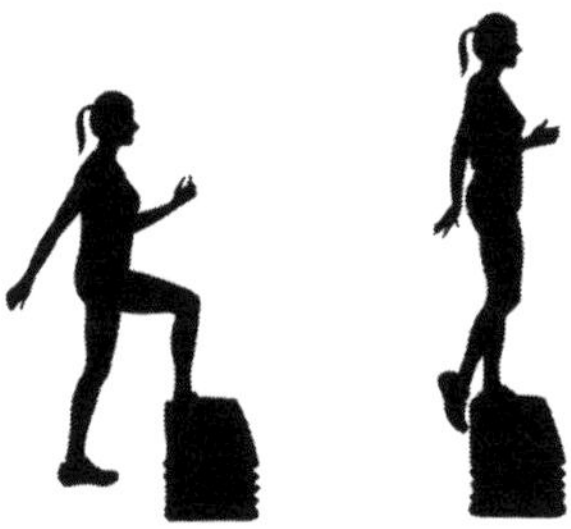

4. Split Squat—Use the stairs in your home or a chair to place one foot behind you. As you lower, your front knee should not go past your toes. You can increase the intensity the further down you go. Start with body weight, and progress to holding weights.

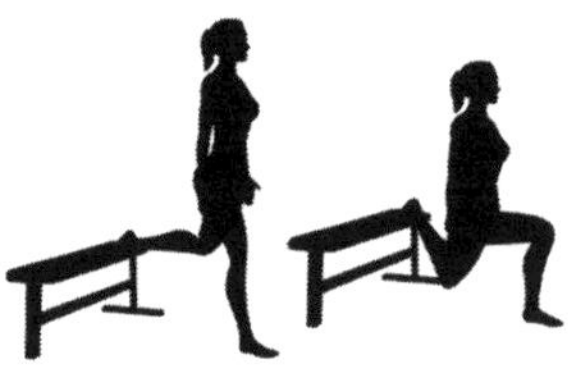

5. Standing Lunges—One of the best exercises for strengthening the glutes and lower leg muscles, lunges involve alternating forward and backward

movements. If you have the space, you can also perform walking lunges, moving back and forth along a hallway or street. Start with body weight, and progress to holding weights.

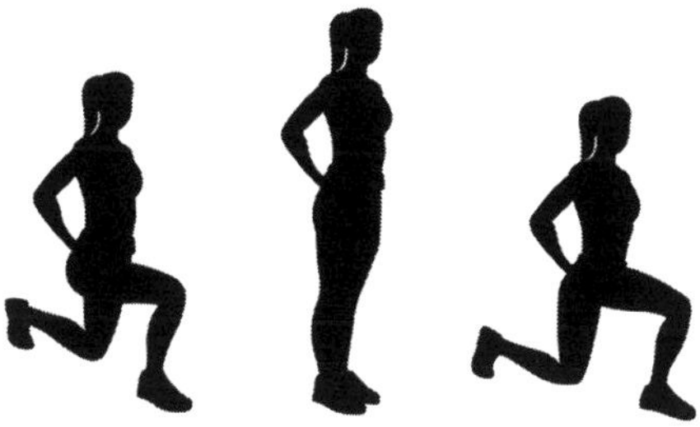

6. Clam Shells—Move down to the floor and lie on your side with your head supported by your hand or arm. Stack your hips and knees. Draw your knees up toward your chest, keeping your ankles together. Lift the top knee toward the sky, holding it there. You can start using your body weight only, and progress to using a band.

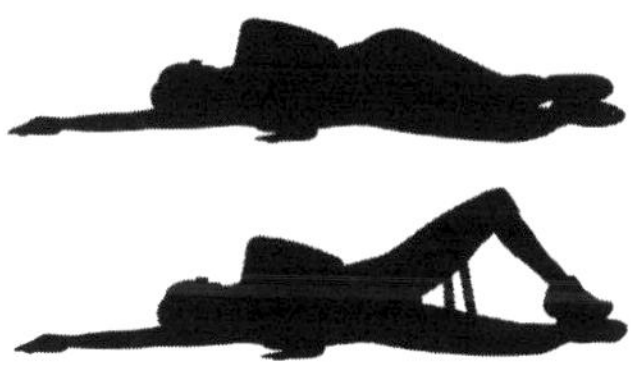

7. Donkey Kicks—Transition to all fours, and keeping your knee bent at a 90-degree angle, contract your glutes and raise the sole of one foot toward the sky. You can start by using your body weight only, and then progress to using a band.

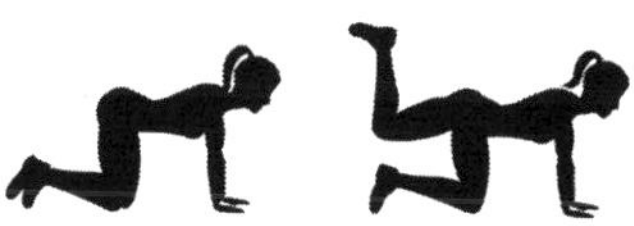

Success Story

Diego was a rectal cancer survivor. He had gone through grueling chemotherapy and was considered cancer-free. He had, though, lost a significant amount of weight from his treatment. His main reason for seeing me was for cancer-related fatigue. He was back to work as a waiter, but found it much more difficult than before to stand on his feet all day.

(Continued)

(Continued)

He used to enjoy hiking, but other than that, he never lifted weights. He started doing yoga, as he had heard that exercise would increase his energy levels. When we looked at his nutritional intake, he consumed a high amount of protein, and he also reported being a good sleeper.

When we assessed his body composition, Diego was found to have very low muscle mass. I stressed the importance of lifting weights, but he couldn't afford a gym membership. I instructed him to perform the exercises above and to buy some inexpensive free weights. He also started doing bicep curls, shoulder presses, and chest presses.

After six weeks, we assessed his body composition, and his muscle mass had increased significantly; most importantly, he had noticed a substantial increase in his energy levels.

References

1 Di Meo S, Napolitano G, Venditti P. Mediators of physical activity protection against ROS-linked skeletal muscle damage. Int J Mol Sci, 2019; 20(12):3024.
2 Tessier A, Wing SS, Rahme E, et al. Association of low muscle mass with cognitive function during a 3-year follow-up among adults aged 65 to 86 years in the Canadian longitudinal study on aging. JAMA Netw Open, 2022; 5(7):e2219926.
3 Walston JD. Sarcopenia in older adults. Curr Opin Rheumatol, 2012; 24(6):623–637.
4 Shachar SS, Deal AM, Weinberg M, et al. Skeletal muscle measures as predictors of toxicity, hospitalization, and survival in patients with metastatic breast cancer receiving taxane-based chemotherapy. Clin Cancer Res, 2017; 23(3):658–65.
5 Chu MP, Lieffers J, Ghosh S, et al. Skeletal muscle density is an independent predictor of diffuse large B-cell lymphoma outcomes treated with rituximab-based chemoimmunotherapy. J Cachexia Sarcopenia Muscle, 2017; 8(2):298–304.
6 Kumar A, Moynagh MR, Multinu F, et al. Muscle composition measured by CT scan is a measurable predictor of overall survival in advanced ovarian cancer. Gynecol Oncol, 2016; 142(2):311–316.
7 Veld J, Vossen JA, De Amorim Bernstein K, et al. Adipose tissue and muscle attenuation as novel biomarkers predicting mortality in patients with extremity sarcomas. Eur Radiol, 2016; 26(12):4649–4655.
8 von Haahling S, Morley JE, Anker SD. An overview of sarcopenia: facts and numbers on prevalence and clinical impact. J Cach Sarc Muscle, 2010; 1:129–133.

9 Lim MT, Pan BJ, Toh DWK, et al. Animal protein versus plant protein in supporting lean mass and muscle strength: a systematic review and meta-analysis of randomized controlled trials. Nutrients, 2021; 13(2):661.

10 Dreyer HC, Drummond MJ, Pennings B, et al. Leucine-enriched essential amino acid and carbohydrate ingestion following resistance exercise enhances mTOR signalling and protein synthesis in human muscle. Am J Physiol Endocrinol Metab, 2008; 294(2):E392–E400.

19

Final Inspiration

You now stand as a true expert on cancer fatigue, understanding it not as an isolated symptom but as a record of the interplay of physical, mental, and emotional forces within your being. This comprehensive perspective is your greatest asset.

The path to overcoming fatigue lies in embracing a holistic approach. No longer will you ignore your body's subtle signals. You've gained invaluable insight into both its normal and imbalanced sensations. You now discern the difference between a fleeting ache and something that may require more attention, empowering you to manage your well-being with newfound clarity.

You are no longer a prisoner to the invisible chains of the mind, nor will you permit anxiety and fear to cast their heavy shadows. Armed with the practice of mindfulness and a host of other tools, you know precisely how to disarm intrusive thoughts and cultivate inner peace.

You understand that movement, whether through vigorous exercise or gentle, restorative motions, is not merely physical activity but a profound catalyst for regaining stamina and strength. Consistently harnessing this power of movement will not only surge your energy but also profoundly refresh your mind.

You are keenly aware that fatigue rarely occurs in isolation. Fatigue infiltrates your social life and relationships, but you recognize that the profound comfort and revitalization found in the presence of friends and loved ones are invaluable, and you value human connection.

You now instinctively gravitate toward the profound nourishment that food offers, prioritizing colorful, nutrient-dense meals as a cornerstone of your daily routine, understanding their vital role in sustaining your energy.

And finally, what could be more holistic and empowering than the power of choice itself? You are no longer a passive bystander simply waiting to feel better but an active participant in your own recovery. You embrace this profound autonomy, free to explore the diverse options now available to you.

Beyond Cancer Fatigue: A Path to Reclaiming Energy, First Edition. Jessa Landmann, ND.

By shifting your perspective and wholeheartedly embracing this holistic approach to cancer-related fatigue, you will navigate its challenges with a newfound strength, armed with a wealth of knowledge. Remember, you are not alone on this journey. You are forging a path toward restoring your energy to such an extent that it will feel as though cancer were truly a thing of the past.

Index

Beyond Cancer Fatigue: A Path to Reclaiming Energy, First Edition. Jessa Landmann, ND.